Bernard
Bringing up our mongol son

Bernard
Bringing up our mongol son

John and Eileen Wilks
Foreword by Olive Stevenson

Routledge & Kegan Paul
London and Boston

First published in 1974
by Routledge & Kegan Paul Ltd
Broadway House, 68-74 Carter Lane,
London EC4V 5EL and
9 Park Street,
Boston, Mass. 02108, USA
Printed in Great Britain by
Northumberland Press Limited
Gateshead

ISBN 0 7100 7791 2 (c)
     0 7100 7792 0 (p)

Contents

Plates

Foreword

There is no doubt that this book will be read eagerly, if not avidly, by those who are involved, as were John and Eileen Wilks, in the upbringing of a mentally handicapped child. For it is well known that the strains inherent in the situation are often enhanced by feelings of isolation. For such parents, this book offers the chance of 'comparing notes' at one remove, of noting differences and similarities and, perhaps most important, of gaining strength from the Wilks's account of their own struggle in what, for any parents, must be a demanding and painful task. They will recognise many of their own reactions in this conspicuously candid and straight-forward account, especially perhaps in those first months of Bernard's life when his 'difference' could not be acknowledged. I have only one reservation about the value of this book to people who are caring for their own handicapped children. John and Eileen Wilks themselves acknowledge that they were in many respects fortunate—in being able to afford an *au pair*, in the fact that Eileen as well as John had an alternative source of satisfaction in academic work and that the day-care facilities in Oxford for Bernard as a child and young adult were very good. They also refer to the value of a larger family unit (seven, including a very impor-tant Granny) in 'spreading the emotional load'.

Thus, whilst in no way minimising the courage, humour and determination which shines through these pages, as well as the typically British understatement (perhaps in consequence the more poignant) of the sad aspects of the story, I should be sorry if others, perhaps less fortunate in their material and practical cir-cumstances or in the solidarity of their family life, were made to feel in any way guilty when they read of the remarkable efforts and success in the development of Bernard's potential. For it is inherent in such situations that parents do feel guilty; at a conscious level, there is the constant nagging question 'have I done enough?' At a deeper level, there is often an irrational, but none the less powerful feeling of guilt that the very condition is in some way 'their fault'. The latter can reinforce the former. The bald fact is that many such parents struggle with well-nigh intolerable conditions of financial hardship and unsuitable housing (a particularly stressful matter). If, on top of that, their marriage or family relationships are less secure than those of the authors, the day-by-day, hour-by-hour tasks involved in the upbringing of their handicapped child may be well-nigh intolerable. I am sure that John and Eileen Wilks would wish to say with me that one needs to extend compassion to oneself as well as to the handicapped person. One can only do as much as one can. Finding those limits, and structuring family life accordingly, is a vital task for the parents if the loving feelings are to be sustained and to grow and the job is not to turn into a barren duty. Having made the point, I must nevertheless reiterate my conviction that the description of the seventeen years of Bernard's life will be a source of much really useful practical information, even advice (especially about firmness in training at certain stages), as well as straightforward relief at the realisation that someone else has been through it too!

I hope, however, that the book will have a much wider readership than this 'inner circle' of parents with a similar problem. For ordinary parents, it can do much to awaken their imagination and sympathy for the task of the parents in such cases. The authors comment on the difficulties which 'outsiders' have in striking a balance between ignoring the existence of the problem and inappropriate curiosity. There is increasing evidence from a variety of studies that the attitude of the general public to disablement of various kinds is confused and ambivalent. The descriptions in this book are paralleled, for example, in accounts of behaviour to blind people, such as asking their *companions* if they take sugar in their tea! The reasons for this are complex: there is a problem of stigma, deriving in part, I believe, from a deepseated fear of the 'abnormal'. There is a problem of social embarrassment, of not knowing the rules of social interaction when confronted with a person who is in some way different. This book is to be welcomed for its frank, common-sensical account of life with Bernard in a wide variety of social contexts, for it should help to dispel some of the myths and

some of the embarrassments. (And it does not deny that Eileen herself was acutely conscious of such embarrassment in the earlier
years.)

For the professionals, whether doctors, social workers or others
in allied occupations, the book is a mine of the kind of detailed
information which is needed if those who visit, advise or counsel,
are genuinely to understand the nature of the daily task. It cannot
be too strongly emphasised that effective social, psychological and
physical help must be based on a practical awareness of just what is
involved in upbringing and care. The great merit of the book (perhaps because its authors are scientists!) is its precision in description. Of course, Bernard is Bernard, not just 'a mongol child', and
one cannot generalise from his characteristics, problems and
achievements to others. For instance, his speech difficulties seem to
have been peculiarly acute and it is possible that this increased the
frequency of tantrums through frustration. But the detail is needed
for this 'imaginative leap' to be made by those who have not lived
with a handicapped child. Furthermore, the more theoretically
inclined will find much to interest them in certain aspects of
child psychology: for example, it is not surprising, but none the
less intriguing, to see how Bernard's anxiety about separation from
his mother extended beyond the age of ordinary children. It is
fascinating to observe his responses to the discipline of his father
and the effectiveness of methods which, although applied in-
tuitively, in fact correspond with current theoretical emphases
in behaviourist psychology. For me, the account of Bernard's
affection for his 80-year-old Granny and hers for him, and of his
capacity for and enjoyment of helping her gives much food for
thought. Does *anyone*, disabled or elderly, want only to be on the
receiving end?

The authors are generous in their praise of the day-care facilities
available for Bernard and their impressions of the local subnormality hospital are also favourable. They are well aware of the
serious criticisms which have been levelled at some such provisions, both in terms of scarcity and, on occasions, shocking in-
adequacies of care in residential institutions. The spotlight is now,
of course, on these deficiencies and there is no doubt that strenuous
efforts are being made to improve conditions and quality of care,
although there is a very long way to go.

Perhaps less attention is being given to the role of the social
worker in relation to families caring for mentally handicapped

persons. Social workers are conspicuous by their absence in this book. The Wilks probably had no need for such, supported as they were by an informed circle of intelligent friends, including doctors and priests. Yet it is, I think, unarguable that for many such families, there is a role for the social worker, to mobilise the available resources and, no less important, to help families find ways of coping with the social and emotional adjustments required of them. I hope this book will find its way on to student social workers' reading lists.

The characteristically unsentimental and matter-of-fact style of the authors makes it essential for me to avoid fulsomeness. But I must conclude by saying that, for me, this book has yet again confirmed my faith in the remarkable human capacity to use, what is, inescapably, a tragedy as an opportunity for the enrichment of family relationships.

Olive Stevenson
Reader in Applied Social Studies
Oxford University

Preface

We have four children, three sons and a daughter. Our second son is a mongol, and scores a low rating in an intelligence test (48 on the Stanford Binet Scale). He is now 17 years old, and lives with us as one of the family. At times, bringing up Bernard has not been too easy. We have written this book to describe our experiences, in the hope that it may be of help to parents of other handicapped children and perhaps of use to workers in the field of mental handicap.

Mentally handicapped children are just as varied in their nature as ordinary children. We once read that 'it is definitely *easy* to teach these children (ie mongols) rules of good behaviour'. This was not our experience, neither, we believe, that of many other parents. Generalisations of this kind are very unhelpful to parents whose children do not conform to the same pattern. We have therefore tried to give a factual account of our own experiences, and hope that other parents will find at least some of our problems relevant to their own.

We have written this book jointly, and began by writing in the first person, saying how 'we' did this and 'we' did that. However, we found that our attempts to make the necessary distinctions between the activities of 'we', 'Eileen', and 'John' soon became very clumsy. We have therefore written our story in the form of a narrative told by John alone.

J. and E. W.

Acknowledgments

We are much indebted to many people who have helped us to bring up Bernard, not least our family and our children. We do not mention them all by name, for they make so long a list that it becomes difficult to know where to draw the line at the end. However, we wish to thank in particular Dr K. W. Lovell, the Rev. Geoffrey Preston OP, Mr I. J. Price, Dr J. M. Stewart, and Miss A. Wallace. We hope that we have made our indebtedness to them and others, including our *au pair* girls, clear in what we have written.

More particularly for help in the preparation of this book, we wish to thank Mr D. A. Purrett and Mr I. J. Price of the Oxford Social Services Department, for showing us facilities in the city, Miss J. Forshaw of the Mabel Prichard School for reading the chapter on the school, Miss C. E. Renfrew of the United Oxford Hospitals for information on Bernard's speech therapy, Dr Rosemary Rue of the Oxford Regional Hospital Board and Mr Kenneth Wright of Borocourt Hospital for arranging a visit to Borocourt, Dr W. G. Harding and Dr Lilian Kerr for showing us facilities in the Borough of Camden, Dr A. C. Stevenson of the Population Genetics Research Unit for advice on genetic aspects and for providing micrographs of our chromosomes, and Mr E. R. Tudor-Davies of the National Association for Mentally Handicapped Children and Miss Elizabeth Osborne of the Institute for Research into Mental Retardation for providing various information.

The manuscript has been read by Dr Olive Stevenson of the Department of Social and Administrative Studies of Oxford University, and by our friends, the late Dr R. Baldick, Dr and Mrs R. H. Kay, Dr and Mrs L. Kochan, and the Rev. and Mrs J. E. Ralphs. We are grateful for their helpful comments.

Chapter 1

A Brother for David

When Bernard was born seventeen years ago, Eileen and I were living in Oxford with our son David and our *au pair* girl Christine. I had come up to the university for two years during the war, and then went away to spend three years working on radar. I returned to Oxford when the war ended, and during the whole time described in this book have been teaching physics at Pembroke College and doing research in the university laboratories.

Eileen is a physicist as well. After spending the war as a meteorological officer in the WAAF, she took a first degree at London University, and then a research degree on optical microscopy at Royal Holloway College. We met in Skye on a climbing holiday organised by my Oxford tutor, and were married in June 1951. Eileen was able to continue her experiments in Oxford, and we lived there by ourselves, very pleasantly, for the next three years.

From the first, we had some fairly fixed ideas about family planning. I am an only child, and Eileen's brother was some years older than her. When we married, we were quite clear that we should have at least two children, so that they could be companions to each other. On the other hand, we also felt that two would very probably be enough. As time went on, we became confirmed in this view. We lived in the upper half of a house divided into two apartments. Our neighbours below were a young surgeon and his wife with their two pretty and agreeable daughters about 2 or 3 years old, differing in age by about a year. We were impressed by the happy way these little girls played together. It seemed an admirable arrangement, and one which we would do well to follow.

Looking back now, with the benefit of hindsight, our views were pretty unrealistic. We never considered if it was really possible to plan our children to a predetermined time-table. We certainly never thought that one of them might be malformed, retarded, or handicapped in any way. We ignored the fact that a number of our friends had children who suffered from physical handicaps of one sort or another. Had we thought about the matter, we would probably have said that these were accidents of life which did not concern us.

Our first son, David, was born in June 1954. Eileen was working in the laboratory until the day before, even though it was quite obvious that David was well on his way. We were pleased to find that we had produced a rather handsome baby. From the first he had a mass of black hair, rosy cheeks, and an agreeable expression. The doctor no doubt regarded him as just another healthy baby, but he was much more to us. Eileen thought him such a good baby that he did not even seem to cry. However, a notebook kept by his sceptical father soon showed that his cries could be heard in at least twenty out of every twenty-four hours.

David was a pleasant attractive baby, and we were proud of him. Even at that time, however, it did occur to at least one of us that we had had precious little control over what sort of baby we had been producing. Naturally enough, Eileen did not waste time on such cynical thoughts. We still remember one evening soon after David's arrival, when we went out for a walk together. We happened to meet the doctor who had looked after Eileen during the confinement.

'How is the young man?' he asked.

'Oh, he's fine,' said Eileen, beaming. 'He's putting on a pound a week.'

The doctor was not unused to babies putting on weight. He smiled.

'You proud mothers, you're all the same, just like fishermen.'

David continued to thrive, and after a few weeks was taken for a National Health inspection at the local clinic. We had no fears that anything was wrong with him, and he passed all the tests with flying colours. At the end of the examination, the doctor in charge said to Eileen:

'Go away and enjoy him.'

This advice seemed very obvious; we did not appreciate its full significance until much later.

The fourth member of our household was Christine. As Eileen

2

wished to continue with her research work, it was necessary to obtain some help about the house, so at the end of August we had been joined by Christine. She was to be the first of a long succession of foreign girls to help in the house, most of them for about a year, although some for much shorter periods. It was our great good fortune to meet Christine at this time. She had come from Bonn in Germany to spend a year learning English. In the end she stayed with us for two and a half years, and then married an Oxford chemist.

At about the same time we left our apartment to move to the house where we live at present. In order that Eileen could carry on with her work while still feeding David, we fitted out one room for her microscope, while a small closet served as a photographic darkroom. Christine came as an *au pair*. She did the washing up, washed the clothes, and cooked lunch for us. Because Eileen was still working we could also pay someone to do a few hours housework each week.

Our household arrangements went well, thanks in large measure to Christine. Her previous experience in Germany with much younger brothers and sisters stood her in good stead. The first time she met Eileen, David provided her with a good opportunity to demonstrate her skill in dealing with dirty nappies. We have since found that although many would-be *au pair* girls have told us that they 'love children' their love sometimes stops short of some necessary but less glamorous chores.

The months passed by, and life went on much as before, except that there were now four of us about the house instead of two. At Christmas and at Easter we managed to have a few days' holiday. David lay in his cot, watched over by Christine, while Eileen and I went walking or climbing in the Lakes or North Wales. Photographs of David taken during the summer show him looking spritely and intelligent, growing bigger and more quizzical. We also have pictures of him with his two grannies, to whom he was the most wonderful child they had seen for a long time.

The second part of our family plan was now going ahead. We had both felt that David should have a brother as soon as possible, so Bernard was expected in November. By the time we left for our summer holiday, he was visibly on his way. Eileen had found so much pleasure in David that she looked forward with great expectation to Bernard, whom she confidently pictured as a second edition of David. I did not cast my expectations quite so firmly, but we were both sure that David was going to have a brother rather than a sister.

Eileen remained in good health and the pregnancy continued normally until November. Possibly the pregnancy was terminated by Eileen and Christine picking the excessive number of quinces loading a tree at the bottom of the garden. Certainly Bernard arrived the next day, two weeks ahead of schedule, after a straightforward labour of five hours. Our family plan now seemed complete, and Eileen still recalls that at the moment of his birth she thought: 'No more for me.'

Eileen's immediate reaction, to herself, on seeing Bernard was: 'Oh, he's not like David.'

He was in fact a rather wizened little fellow, with a slightly yellowish complexion, but with plenty of black hair. Although not much different from many other babies we had seen before, he was quite clearly not as cherubic as David. His birth weight of 7¼ lb. although satisfactory was not as noteworthy as his elder brother's 8½ lb.

Although Bernard looked quite different from David, we never suspected that anything was wrong. After two days he was still somewhat yellow, so the midwife took him away for an inspection at the hospital. He came back after two hours; a test had shown that no jaundice was present, and the yellow colour went in a few days. However, Eileen had to spend a long time feeding him; he was inept at sucking and dribbled inordinately. This was an ominous sign, but one which we did not appreciate at the time. Meanwhile the quinces, picked from the garden, ripened in the kitchen, and their sweet smell began to pervade the house.

Bernard soon showed that he had his good points. He was a contented little baby, and cried very little. After only ten days he was ready to do without his 2 o'clock feed, and slept quietly all through the night. This again was not really a good sign, but we saw no cause to worry. There was certainly no objection from Eileen, who was always reluctant to turn out of bed in the middle of the night.

Although Bernard soon agreed to be fed at reasonable times, the feeding itself was not so satisfactory. After her experience with David, Eileen thought that she was now expert in the not too difficult art of breast-feeding. Yet in spite of all her efforts, Bernard dribbled, and made an awful mess. To mop up the milky flood, Eileen had to reinforce his ordinary bibs with thick nappies. When

4

she asked the midwife about this dribbling, she was told, 'Some babies are like that.'

David, at least, seemed well pleased with his new brother. He would sit happily on Eileen's lap while she fed Bernard. Eileen had been at home the whole time, so David had not felt put out by the newcomer, and accepted Bernard without any fuss. Probably because David was around, Eileen did not worry too much about Bernard's messy feeding habits during the daytime, but evening feeds were a different matter.

Eileen had always fed David in front of me, but she was reluctant to show me what a messy business it was with Bernard. She had to work quite hard for about an hour in order to give him an adequate meal. Even so, she did not raise the matter of dribbling again with the nurse. Neither did she pay too much attention to his slow increase in weight. He was alive, not crying, he looked all right. Why worry?

Reading this account, it must seem that we were very unperceptive parents. Yet at the time it was not so clear. Our friends duly admired Bernard, and it was only later that two of them admitted that they had thought him 'a funny little baby'. At the beginning of December Christine had called him a 'model baby' because there was no crying. Both his grannies came to stay with us at Christmas, and noticed nothing amiss. The sister at the local clinic who saw Bernard from time to time also said nothing.

Bernard was certainly not as handsome as our elder son, but then we had been particularly impressed by David. Bernard was not really very different from many other babies. Admittedly there was a lack of any feeling of exhilaration over our new son, but then a repeat performance is seldom as exciting as the first occasion. Yet we did not think much about this, for we had plenty to do. We had to give David as much attention as before in order to compensate for the presence of the baby. It was soon Christmas, and all the various tasks involved kept us busy.

Looking back, now, we can see that we almost certainly had hidden reservations. We have built up over the years a series of photographs which give a fairly complete record of our children's progress. Yet it is only quite recently that we realised we had taken no photographs of Bernard until he was about a year old. We have several pictures of our other children taken in their first month or so, but none of Bernard at that age, even though everything was supposed to be in order. We also find that we have not kept any records of his weight, as we did for his brothers and sister.

Possibly we were more disappointed in his appearance than we cared to admit, even to ourselves. Weeks later, two of our friends, who had talked with me on the day that Bernard was born, told Eileen that they had thought from my manner that something was wrong. Certainly I did not feel this consciously. Maybe I was just tired, as I had been up nearly all the previous night, but perhaps I was also disappointed as well.

One day when Bernard was about 6 weeks old, while Eileen was nursing him, she was struck by the appearance of his eyes, which looked very vacant. The thought occurred to her:

'Surely he's not an idiot?'

She put the suggestion aside and did not mention the episode to anyone.

In spite of these hidden undertones, we put Bernard's name down for the same prep school as his brother David. He was then about 2 months old, and as far as we can remember, we made these arrangements without any hesitation at all.

Chapter 2

Bernard

The first clear sign that something was seriously wrong with Bernard came early in the New Year, when he was taken to the local clinic for a routine National Health inspection. By chance, the doctor in charge was a friend of ours, Keith Lovell. Keith began by looking at Bernard in a casual manner, but soon his inspection became much slower, and much more detailed. Eileen began to worry.

'What are you looking at?' she asked anxiously. Keith's reply was not altogether reassuring. 'Oh, these patterns on his hands are rather interesting,' he said, and did not elaborate further.

A day or so later, about tea-time, there was a knock on the front door. Eileen opened it to find our family doctor on the step. She was surprised to see Dr Stewart, for no one was ill, and she was certainly not happy to hear that he had come to see Bernard. After quite a short examination, Dr Stewart explained that there had been a question of jaundice when he was born, but that now he seemed all right. This did not appear to be very important, for as Eileen recalled, the suspected jaundice had cleared up within a few days of birth. However, as she was letting Dr Stewart out, he said that he would like a consulting paediatrician to see Bernard.

'What's wrong, then?' asked Eileen.

'Well,' said Dr Stewart, 'there's something about the eyes we don't like.'

He then left. Eileen shut the door, in tears, for she realised that this indicated some mental trouble. However she recovered herself, as she had to return to the nursery to play with David and Bernard.

The following evening Dr Stewart called again when I was at home. He told us that if Bernard were his own child he would like a second opinion on him. We readily agreed. We were also considerably impressed by the fact that Dr Stewart was looking much more serious than usual. Although nothing very specific was said that evening, both of us by then were fairly clear that Bernard was going to be mentally backward in some way or other.

A few days later Dr Stewart came back with the consulting paediatrician. The two doctors examined Bernard in our presence, and then retired to compare notes. On their return, the paediatrician explained that there were indeed grounds for concern, and that Bernard would need some special attention. As far as we can now remember, not much more was said on this occasion. However, it was quite clear to both of us that our suspicions about mental backwardness were fully justified.

The following day, Eileen took Bernard to the local clinic, and had a talk with the sister in charge.

'Oh, yes,' she said, 'he's a mongol. I've thought so for a long time.'

The word 'mongol' would not have meant anything to me, but to Eileen it was a very formidable word. She knew exactly what it meant, for she had grown up with a mongol girl, a few years older, living in the same street. This girl, Nina, could talk moderately well, but one look at her face was enough to show that she was very backward mentally. She could find her own way to school, but once there she remained at the back of the bottom form, and was ignored all day. Most of the children and neighbours had been kind to her, but Eileen knew that her parents had very seldom invited Nina into their house.

Eileen accepted the sister's sympathy with some composure, and returned home, pushing Bernard in his pram. Christine had taken David out for a walk, so for the next hour the house was empty. It began to sink in that Bernard was going to be like Nina, whom Eileen had always thought of as an 'idiot'. She was appalled by the realisation that one of her own children would be no better than Nina. She did not want to accept the fact. She did not want to think about Nina, in the hope that maybe the nightmare would go away. Yet in her innermost heart she did not doubt that the sister was right about Bernard. The future seemed very bleak, and feeling very sorry for herself she sat down and cried.

Eileen had now been carrying Bernard for nine months, and feeding him herself for three months. Now she had to face the fact that she had produced an 'idiot'. She realised that for a long time

Bernard would have to be taken about, and that people in the street would stare at him, and worse still at her. She would have to admit to everybody that her own son, not somebody else's, but her own son, was an 'idiot'.

Alone in the nursery, life appeared very hard, and Eileen wept bitterly with Bernard lying there peacefully in his cot. As time went on, she began to feel sorry for him, for this poor little fellow who would always be helpless in the face of the world. She prayed for strength to be able to face up to the world herself, and to accept Bernard as he was. Yet, at that moment at least, she did not want to accept Bernard as being a mongol. She still did not want to accept the sister's diagnosis as correct. She hoped that perhaps the doctors would tell us a different story, so she decided not to tell me anything about Nina.

Eventually Christine and David returned home. Eileen pulled herself together, so that she could behave normally in front of David. She played with him, fed Bernard with David on her lap as usual, and then put David to bed. When I came home we had supper with Christine, and it was not until after supper, when we were alone, that she told me what the sister had said. She was vague as to what the term 'mongol' implied, although we were both clear that some fairly drastic form of mental backwardness was involved. Keith Lovell had told us that he would come round the next evening to explain matters in more detail, so we decided to wait and see what he would say. We then went off to the cinema as already arranged, and did not discuss the matter much further.

The prospect seemed no brighter when we woke up in the morning. We were certainly very depressed. Trying to recall my feelings at the time, I am pretty sure that I was not excessively worried that Bernard would not win prizes or scholarships, or achieve any of those things which parents are traditionally proud of. I had already seen fathers make both themselves and their sons miserable by expecting too much, and by trying to push their children beyond their natural capacities.

I was not much concerned because I would not be able to tell my friends what a clever son I had. I was, however, extremely depressed by the prospect of the sheer disorganisation and disturbance that seemed to be involved. Bernard would almost certainly have to be looked after indefinitely. We would never be able to leave him alone in the house, and he would be a considerable burden and responsibility whenever we took him out. He would never fit in with all the various activities one hopes to do with one's family.

Eileen went off to the laboratory as usual. She concentrated on her work there, and talked to people as if nothing had happened. In fact she hardly thought about Bernard all morning. However, when she came back to the house at lunch-time, it was a different matter.

That evening Keith Lovell came round to tell us something about mongolism. Eileen still did not reveal that she was quite knowledge-able on this subject already. Keith said that mongols can be recog-nised by characteristic patterns in the lines on their hands, as well as by their slanted eyes, sloping up and outwards. We were to realise later that the typical mongoloid face is very easily recog-nised, provided one knows what to look for. As a further but less obvious means of identification, the big toe is generally far more separated from the other toes than is the case in normal children.

We were told that mongols are generally more susceptible to illnesses than ordinary children, particularly to chest complaints. Quite often they suffer from heart disorders. As a result, relatively trivial illnesses like mumps or measles may affect them seriously, and in the past many mongols have died from various ailments in their first few years. As a result their expectation of life was much reduced, but nowadays many live to the age of fifty or more.

The medical examination had shown that Bernard was quite healthy. His heart was sound, and there was no sign of any other physical ailments. It was too early to tell what we might expect for his eventual mental age. Mongols vary considerably in this respect, but an optimistic average seemed to be somewhat less than ten years.

It became clear that there was not a great deal that could be done for Bernard immediately. Indeed the main difference between him and other children seemed to be that he would grow up much more slowly. Armed with this somewhat depressing knowledge, we could only wait and see.

During the next week Dr Stewart called to see us. He told us that all the doctors had suspected that Bernard was a mongol soon after he was born. He himself had not been quite sure, and had hopefully argued the other way because Eileen's eyes slanted slightly. However this was only a vague hope, because he had also wondered why we ourselves had not realised that Bernard was so unlike David. The doctors had been waiting for us to realise that all was not well, and were somewhat mystified that we had not called on them to seek advice. Maybe we were unobservant. Maybe we should have taken notice of several warning signs which we put aside. However, a willingness to take what comes without too much questioning was to stand us in good stead in the future.

Chapter 3

Advice

During his visit to us, Keith Lovell had tried to give us some idea of the sort of person that Bernard would become. Mongols are in fact a well-defined type, and it is possible to get a fairly accurate picture of their likely behaviour. However, they tend to live rather out of sight, in their homes or schools, so most people know little about them.

Keith was not altogether reassuring. He explained to us that mongols are invariably very affectionate and lovable. On the other hand they were sometimes what he called 'destructive'. We did not follow up this point too closely; in any case Keith did not seem to have any very precise information.

We learnt that, in those days, there were two types of schools for the mentally backward. First of all there were the ESN, or Educationally Subnormal, schools for those children whose intelligence fell just below the limit of what was required for attendance at ordinary schools. It was also made clear to us that Bernard might have so low an intelligence that he would not make the grade for an ESN school, but would have to go to what was then called an occupation centre. Although a few mongols had sufficient ability to profit from the teaching at the ESN schools, most of them attended the occupation centres.

We were particularly anxious to know the answer to one question: 'Will he grow up to look as if there is something wrong with him?' We felt that even if he was a little weak in the head, it would be more bearable if it were not too obvious. Keith gave another of his noncommittal replies, and said that he would arrange for us to visit an ESN school where we could see children aged between 5 and 16 years.

Some days later we went to the ESN school, and were very kindly received by the headmaster. He told us of the work the school was doing, and of the training the pupils received, and then took us round the various classrooms. We were much impressed by the care and devotion of the teachers, but saw little else to encourage us. The children were all clearly below par, even though they were probably more intelligent than Bernard. The school itself was housed in a collection of old huts, in fair enough condition, but not really very attractive in decoration or equipment. Since then there have been big improvements, but of course we were not to know that. We returned home in a rather sombre mood.

Although we had little enthusiasm for the ESN school, we were fairly clear that Bernard was probably not good enough for it. However, no one suggested to us that we should visit the occupation centre, where Bernard was most likely to go. In any case we had been so disheartened by the ESN school that we had no particular desire to make the visit. Bernard was still only 3 months old, so there was no need for hurry.

Rather to our surprise, we now began to receive advice from several quarters. Looking back, we are most grateful that so much of this advice was both kind and to the point. We began to learn that some form of mental handicap among children is not at all uncommon. When Bernard was born we knew almost nothing of the various mental disabilities that may be present in children. We had never had any reason to be interested, and in those days there was much less discussion of these matters in public and in the press.

Our first reaction to the diagnosis was that this was so awful that life would never be the same again. However, we soon realised that Bernard was by no means unique. A friend told us that one of his sisters, although not a mongol, had been handicapped in a similar way. We were introduced to a doctor living little more than a hundred yards away who had a mongol daughter about 8 years old.

It soon became clear that some of our friends knew considerably more about mongols and mental handicap than we did, and had clear ideas as to what should be done. The best advice came from Dr Stewart and from my professor at the laboratory, Sir Francis Simon. Dr Stewart's recommendation was quite clear and unambiguous: 'The best thing you can do is to have another baby.'

This turned out to be the easiest advice to put into practice, and

13

just over a year later Bernard was joined by a brother, Andrew Simon.

Sir Francis, one of the kindliest men we have known, and also one of the wisest, knew all about mongols and mental backwardness. His wide circle of acquaintances included several friends and colleagues whose children had been handicapped in one way or another. He impressed on me that it was most important that we should not let our other children suffer because of Bernard. It might therefore be best, in time, to send Bernard away to a home.

Shortly afterwards we talked with the doctor and his wife living near us, who had a mongol daughter in addition to three other children, both older and younger. The mongol girl was then 8 years old, and stayed indoors most of the time. We gathered that the parents' main cause for concern arose from the interactions between the girl and her brothers and sisters. She did not want to play with them much, principally because she could not keep up with them. Relationships had become strained when the younger children had 'grown through' the mental age of the handicapped child. The youngest daughter had found this time particularly difficult; she had become rather troublesome, and somewhat spiteful towards her mongol sister.

Keith Lovell also arranged for Eileen to meet the mother of a mongol girl aged fourteen who attended the ESN school. This lady very kindly invited Eileen to her home, where she had tea with the mongol daughter and her normal sister aged sixteen. Afterwards, Eileen was shown family photographs of the girl as she had grown up. It was very obvious, both from looking at the photographs and from meeting the girl, that one could not conceal the fact that one's child was a mongol.

Eileen saw that the mother was extremely fond of her mongol daughter. The girl was able to do various jobs about the house, and her mother remarked that she was more helpful than her normal 16-year-old. Eileen remembers that the 16-year-old was present at the time, and (not surprisingly) seemed to resent the remark. It was again clear that care would be needed to avoid serious difficulties between a mongol and his normal brothers and sisters.

We also recall two other conversations. Eileen's parish priest was most sympathetic and kind, as indeed he always had been ever since she had known him. However, he did not provide us with any specific advice. A friend arranged for us to talk to an acquaintance who had similar problems in his own family. It turned out that he had three or four children, and was deeply troubled by two of them; one child had to attend an ESN school, and another had just failed to obtain a scholarship at a well-known public school. We were impressed that the failure to get the scholarship seemed as heavy a burden to the father as the difficulties of the child at the ESN school.

We were much struck by the number of times we were told that mongols are most likely to be born to intelligent parents. Living in a university town, we do in fact know several gifted people with handicapped children. It is also quite clear from visiting special schools and training centres that the incidence of mongolism is spread pretty evenly throughout the community.

Why was this remark about intelligence made so often? There is undoubtedly a belief, seldom consciously formulated but deeply rooted, that idiot children come from idiot parents. This may be true of some forms of mental backwardness, but it is certainly not true in general, and certainly not true of mongols. Eileen and I were always aware of this fact, and in any case our university degrees assured us that we were of normal intelligence. We did not worry over this point. Yet the existence of this subconscious attitude was made very clear to us, and probably makes an unnecessary burden for many parents of handicapped children.

At no stage did we feel inclined to query the medical diagnosis. Bernard had been examined by our own doctor, by Keith Lovell, and by a consulting paediatrician, as well as by the sister at the clinic. They were all unanimous in their opinion. We had also talked with Eileen's cousin, a consulting neurologist. His view was that if a child had been diagnosed as a mongol, it was a waste of time to query the decision, because it was not at all easy to be wrong. He also said: 'It's a miracle that any baby is born without some defect.'

We would have found the diagnosis hard to accept if it had been pronounced on our previous child David. However, we probably already had some unconscious reservations, and the judgment seemed only too reasonable. Nothing was to be gained by arguing the point further.

Looking back, I think that it is true to say that we accepted nearly all the advice we received, and acted on the greater part of it. Only on one point does Eileen now feel that the picture was not altogether complete. It so happened that all the parents we talked to had mongol daughters rather than sons, and they were all described as having a placid nature. As time has shown, the word 'placid' has seldom been a suitable description of Bernard. Yet no great harm was done by our not learning immediately that we were in for a certain amount of trouble!

As the years have gone by, we have come to know an increasing number of handicapped children and their parents. These contacts, especially the early ones, helped us enormously for two reasons. We learned that although Bernard would never go to an ordinary school, there was a considerable organisation of special schools and training centres where he would be looked after, and helped to develop what abilities he had to the best advantage. It was also apparent that at least some of the parents were not unduly, or even at all, bowed down by their responsibilities.

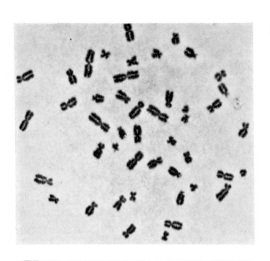

1a Picture of chromo-
somes: John Wilks

1b Picture of chromo-
somes: John Wilks

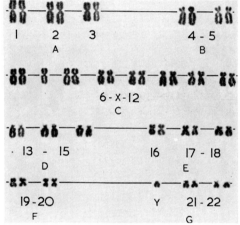

1   2   3   4 - 5
      A   B

6 - X - 12
C

13 - 15   16   17 - 18
    D   E

19 - 20   Y   21 - 22
   F   G

1c Picture of chromo-
somes: Bernard
Wilks

1   2   3   4 - 5
      A   B

6 - X - 12
C

13 - 15   16   17 - 18
    D   E

19 - 20   Y   21 - 22
   F   G

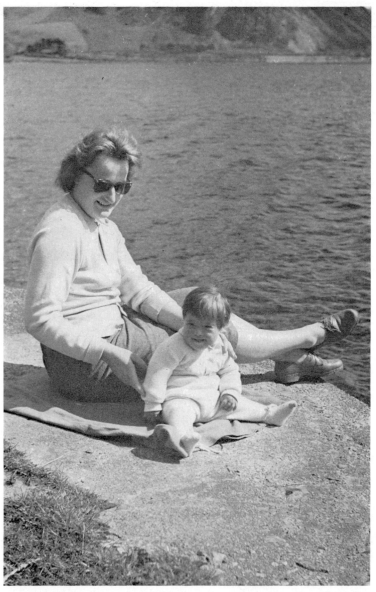

2 Our earliest photograph of Bernard, aged 16 months, with Cilli.
A happier picture than the blank expression in *Plate 3* taken three
months later

Chapter 4

About Mongolism

Before going on with our story of Bernard, I think it will be useful to give a short account of what the doctors can now tell us about mongolism, and why Bernard is different from other children. It has been known for a long time that mongols have some very characteristic physical features. They tend to be short in stature, with round heads, and eyes which slant upwards and outwards. This slant of the eyes gives them a characteristic Chinese or Mongol appearance, which once perceived is readily recognised on future occasions. They tend to have large tongues, and are apt to go about with their mouth open. There are also many other detailed physical differences associated with mongolism, but most of these are quite technical and I only mention one more.

It has been known for over thirty years that the patterns of lines on hands and feet of mongols differ appreciably from those of normal people. To put the matter more colloquially, mongols can be identified by their fingerprints. This immediately suggests that, whatever the nature of the defect responsible for mongolism, the defect enters very deeply into the whole structure of the mongol. Moreover the defect is present from a very early stage of development, because the characteristic fingerprints of mongolism are known to be developing in the infant foetus only ten weeks after conception.

It has always seemed very clear to us that, because the signs of mongolism are so all-pervading, there is very little chance of finding any treatment or medicine to remedy the condition. Mongolism is not a case of the human machine working incorrectly, but of a human machine having grown up differently in the first place. It follows that there is at present no medical treatment which can turn a mongol into a normal child. Neither is there likely to be.

When Bernard was born, we were told that mongolism was not hereditary, but appeared to be the result of some random accident or misfortune, which statistics showed to occur once in about every 600 births. The only factor which appeared to influence the likelihood of a mongol birth was the age of the parents. On the average, for mothers under 30 years of age, 1 birth in every 1,000 would be a mongol. This figure rose to 1·5 per 1,000 for mothers aged between 30 and 34, to 3 per 1,000 for mothers between 35 and 39, and 10 per 1,000 for mothers between 40 and 45. For older parents the chances increased still more rapidly. These figures clearly suggest that mongolism is some accident arising from the natural processes of ageing. We were advised, after Bernard's birth that as far as could be seen the incidence of mongolism was quite random. In fact, there were suggestions in the medical literature that possibly in a very small number of cases mongolism did run in families. However, the evidence was by no means clear, and in any case the incidence of this hereditary or familial mongolism was very low. Therefore from a practical point of view we were given the right information. Since then, considerable advances have been made in the study of mongolism, and these views have had to be slightly modified.

The first recognition of mongolism as a distinct condition was made in 1866 when Dr Langdon Down described a condition which he called mongolian idiocy. Since then the condition has been given a variety of names, of which the best known are mongolism, Down's anomaly, and Down's syndrome. (An anomaly is an unusual condition. A syndrome is a collection of symptoms, a convenient expression for a condition like mongolism which had many symptoms but no well-understood cause.) Since Dr Down's first paper, there has been an increasing number of publications studying all aspects of mongolism. Most of these are scientific papers written for doctors, and the general reader will find them rather hard going. Those interested will find a good summary of this work in the book *Down's Anomaly* by Dr L. S. Penrose and Dr G. F. Smith. These scientific investigations are of great importance for our ultimate understanding of mongolism, but we have to admit that most of them do not give much immediate practical advice to parents of mongol children. There is however one exception, a relatively recent development, which concerns the hereditary aspects of mongolism.

To explain this new development, we must first describe one or two aspects of modern biology. All living matter is made up from what are called cells. These cells are extremely small, certainly less than one-thousandth of an inch in diameter, and are invisible to the naked eye. Nevertheless, using ordinary microscopes, we can obtain pictures of them the size of a snapshot. As most of the cells are very transparent, a direct picture of them shows very little detail. However, if the cell is stained with coloured dyes, different parts of the cell take up the dyes preferentially, and become visible because of their different colours. This technique shows that the cell, although extremely small, contains within its walls a large number of different constituents. By a suitable choice of dyes, all the various constituents can be clearly seen under the microscope. Further study reveals that a cell consists of a distinct central region, or nucleus, surrounded by other material called the cytoplasm. Both the nucleus and cytoplasm show further structure.

Let us now turn to the process of growth in living matter. Any animal or plant is built up from a vast number of cells. When the animal or plant grows, it does so, not by each cell becoming bigger, but by the number of cells increasing. A cell has the power to reproduce itself, and all growth takes place by single cells splitting into two, thus giving rise to two completely new cells of the same type. This growth by division is a very complex matter. Cells in the different parts of our body, the muscle, the brain, the heart, the liver, are all different in type, and it is essential that when they divide into two, the new cells are of exactly the right form for their particular location.

The cell is a remarkable entity, besides being able to reproduce itself, it is all the while a living organism. If it is a muscle cell, it has the power of converting the energy in our blood into muscular force. If it is a liver cell, it is a miniature chemical factory to regulate the running of the body. When we take a photograph of a nucleus, using suitable dyes, we see a large number of threadlike substances known as *chromosomes* (*Plate 1a*). Different plants and different animals have different numbers of chromosomes, but as a general rule all plants and animals of the same species have the same number of chromosomes. These chromosomes can be identified and arranged in groups, as shown in *Plate 1b*, and the characteristic arrangement of the chromosomes is the same for each species of plant or animal.

There is now very good evidence that the chromosomes contain

virtually all the information needed to ensure that the minute ferti-
lised egg of a mother grows up to be an animal of the same type as
its parents, and with physical and mental traits characteristic of its
parents. The chromosomes are in fact a vast store of information, a
blueprint for the final living plant or animal. The chromosomes are
minute, magnified a thousand times they are little more than one-
tenth of an inch long, as in *Plate 1*. How then can they be a vast
store of information? We must remember that although very small
to the eye, the chromosomes contain a tremendous number of
atoms, which can be arranged in a fantastically large number of
ways. These different arrangements of the atoms correspond to the
vast variety of life in the plant and animal world, and to the
wide range of human physique and personality.

It is important to realise that all animals begin their existence
as one single cell, with one set of chromosomes, which is formed
following the union of the parents. Therefore the chromosomes in
this cell contain the whole information for the future development
of the animal. To produce the full-grown animal, this one cell will
divide many times, and in doing so will produce different types of
cell to build up the muscles, the bones, the brain, etc. Yet at each
division, the chromosomes of the new cells are an exact replica
of those of the old. Thus all the vast number of cells in our bodies
contain the same number of identical chromosomes.

We have said that the chromosomes are a tremendously complicated array of vast numbers of atoms. How then does this complicated arrangement duplicate itself exactly each time a cell divides
into two? Without going into any details, we can say that this
duplication is made possible because the chromosomes are con-
structed from their atoms in a special way. This special arrangement permits the chromosome to act as a template, so that under
the appropriate conditions, a second identical chromosome can
be grown side by side with the first. When this operation has
been completed, the new double chromosome splits along its length,
giving two chromosomes identical to the first. Thus there are now
two identical chromosomes, one for each new cell.

All normal human cells contain 46 chromosomes, which may be
grouped in 23 pairs. Moreover, because these chromosomes are of
different lengths and of somewhat different shape, it is possible to
allocate numbers to them to indicate the different types, as shown
in *Plate 1b*. It was discovered about ten years ago that all mongols
appear to have an extra number-21 chromosome, or at least the

major part of one. This may be either quite separate from the other number-21 chromosomes, as in *Plate 1c*, or possibly attached to another chromosome. Hence, as we had surmised, mongolism is a defect built into the very structure of an individual.

We have already said that chromosomes reproduce themselves exactly. If this is so, how does a mongol have an extra chromosome when his parents are normal? The answer is that occasionally something goes wrong when a cell grows into two cells. It seems that most forms of mongolism arise from some mistake in a process which we must now explain. We have said that normal people have grown from a single cell containing 46 chromosomes. Yet this single cell was originally formed by the union of a male and a female cell. Male and female cells each in general have 46 chromosomes, why then does the resulting single cell not have a total of 92 chromosomes? The answer is that the sex cells in their last stages in the parent's bodies, undergo a special process. That is, they divide in such a way that each final cell contains only 23 chromosomes, so that the act of conception brings together two cells each with 23 chromosomes. This division process is known as *meiosis*, and it seems that mongolism usually arises at this stage of development. It appears that some malfunctioning occurs with the result that, after the division process, one of the final cells contains an extra chromosome. It then follows irrevocably that a child formed from this cell will have a total of 47 chromosomes. This situation is responsible for Bernard's condition, and for most cases of mongolism. It is known as *trisomy*, and accounts for about 96 per cent of all mongolism. We now turn to some of the remaining cases.

Sometimes the cell may contain the extra number-21 chromosome, characteristic of mongolism, attached to another chromosome. Although there are now only 46 separate chromosomes, one of them is extra large, and the child is again a mongol. The importance of this 46-chromosome or *translocate* type of mongolism is that it seems to arise when an apparently normal parent has chromosomes that are actually somewhat different from normal. The parent in question is said to be a *translocate carrier* of mongolism. Just as for defects such as haemophilia, there is the possibility that the child of a carrier may be a mongol. In fact the probability of the child being a mongol may be as high as 1 in 3. Although cases of translocate mongolism are rare, they are of importance because the chromosome defect in the parent may have been transmitted to the apparently normal brothers and sisters of a mongol child. These brothers and sisters are then liable to produce mongol children.

There are several other possibilities, of which we only mention one, namely that an apparently normal parent may be what is termed *mosaic*. That is, although the majority of his cells have 46 chromosomes, some have 47. This would be the result of errors somewhere along the chain of the reproductive process. In general the 46-chromosome cells predominate and the parent appears normal. However, there is a chance that a child may be formed from a 47-chromosome cell, in which case he would be a mongol. The amount of mosaicism may vary from virtually no 47-chromosome cells to a substantial fraction. It follows that the probability of a mongol child being born is greater than for normal parents, but less than for pure translocate parents. The actual probability can only be estimated by a detailed consideration of the particular chromosomes in question, but in general comes out to figures in the range between 1 in 10 and 1 in 20. Like translocate mongolism, mosaicism may be passed down from parents to their apparently normal children.

We have now gone far enough in trying to describe what may be a very complicated situation. To sum up, we can say that mongolism is now firmly related to a defect in the number and arrangements of the chromosomes in the cell. Usually both parents are quite normal, and the mongol has an extra separate chromosome. These cases are known as trisomy and there is not much risk of another child being a mongol. In a few other cases, such as translocate mongolism and mosaicism, the source of the trouble lies in the chromosomes of the parents. Although the parents themselves may be apparently normal, the probability of another mongol being born to them, and to their apparently normal children, may be considerable. In any case, an estimate of the probabilities can be made by an examination of the chromosomes in the cells of the child and the parents.

These details were not fully appreciated when Bernard was born, but today they should always be taken into account by parents, and their advisers, when considering whether to have further children.

Besides being mentally retarded, mongols also tend to suffer from a wide range of physical ailments (although Bernard seems to be rather an exception). They are unduly liable to various infections of the lungs, and alimentary canal, and sometimes have serious heart defects. They are susceptible to minor ailments such as catarrh, dental troubles, chilblains, etc. Yet these various physical disabilities are similar to those of normal children, and need treating in just the same way. The mongol only differs from the normal child in that he has an unfair share of these ailments. As a result, the expectation of life for mongols has hitherto been very low, not more than about ten years, which means of course that many died much younger. However, the position today is changing because the use of modern drugs to overcome infection ensures the survival of many more of these children. We may therefore expect to see an increasing number of mongols growing up to an advanced age.

Fortunately, Bernard has managed to avoid the various physical disabilities that often go with mongolism, the weak chest, the heart defects, and the runny nose. He has always been a very healthy child. He has run through the usual childish ailments of mumps, measles and chickenpox, but he was never really ill with any of them. We are also fortunate in that Bernard has a small appetite, and knows when he's had enough. On the other hand, when some of his friends used to come to tea, they often seemed unable to stop eating. Not surprisingly they were often rather fat and puffy. Admittedly Bernard is prepared to eat sweets and chocolate in sufficient quantity to make himself ill, but this is usually avoided by careful rationing.

Chapter 5

Growing Up. The First Five Years

The first year

Bernard's progress during his first year was fairly uneventful. We expect a normal baby to do very little for his first three months; he spends his time being fed, bathed, and returned to sleep in his cot. Then he gradually moves on to the next stage, and becomes a real person. He starts to take an interest in everything around him, he investigates himself, discovers his toes; plays with his rattle or a woolly ball. For the whole of his first year, Bernard did none of these things.

He never touched a rattle, or took an interest in anything. He was content just to eat and sleep. He made none of the many experiments a normal child makes in trying to do things for the first time. David had tried to sit up at an early age, and had become annoyed and angry when he found this too difficult for him. Bernard had no such ambitions, and remained quite calm and unfrustrated. Except for the difficulties of feeding him, he was no trouble at all. He hardly ever cried, and lay quietly in his pram. Eventually he had to be encouraged to sit up, so we began by propping him against a pile of cushions. He never made any dramatic attempt to sit up on his own, but as the months went by he needed less and less propping, until finally he was able to sit unaided.

When we learnt that Bernard was a mongol, Dr Stewart advised Eileen to stop feeding him at her breast, lest certain unspecified psychological difficulties arose. This was one piece of advice which Eileen did not take. Her motives were mixed. She was sorry for Bernard, he was deprived enough as it was, why should he be still further deprived? Breast-feeding also seemed much less trouble, without all the routine work involved in filling and cleaning bottles. Even so, each feed took almost an hour, and it was hard work with little pleasure in it.

Eileen continued to feed Bernard until he was about six months old when she weaned him on to Farex, a porridge-like material. The procedure, to put it crudely, was to push the food into him with a spoon. This was a slow and messy business, but not too difficult. Drinking presented more problems, as it was quite impossible to make use of an ordinary cup. At first he was fed milk with a spoon relatively easily. We also experimented with various types of unspillable beakers, but it was a long time before these were of much assistance.

It was at meal times that Bernard showed the first signs of a characteristic personality. Shortly after beginning on Farex, Eileen decided to give him a more varied diet, with the usual proteins of meat and eggs. These were utterly and completely rejected. We soon found out that he was absolutely opposed to eating any form of solid food except mashed banana. This did not seem to make for a very balanced diet, but he was willing to accept protein in the form of chocolate mixed in the banana, and we spooned orange juice into him separately. We therefore reminded ourselves that he was also getting milk with the Farex, and did not bother too much about his diet. One of the city health visitors called to see Eileen every two or three months. She had had no previous experience of a mongol, and was somewhat nonplussed by the banana and chocolate diet. She had no suggestions to make, only remarking 'Well, he's still alive'.

We kept no detailed records of Bernard's progress. Therefore, in recalling how he progressed from month to month, we find it helpful to recall him as he was on holidays and excursions, which stand out as milestones in the year. At Easter we all stayed in a cottage at Chapel Farm in the Lake District, and we have pictures of David chasing ducks in the field outside. Bernard spent the time quietly in the carry-cot inside the cottage, looked after by Christine who also kept an eye on David. (It was no hardship for Christine not to come out walking with us, as she had very carefully brought only high-heeled shoes up to the Lakes.) At Whitsuntide my mother came to spend a week with us at Oxford. We have happy pictures of her with David and Christine in the garden. Bernard presumably was still flat on his back in the pram.

For our summer holiday we all went to Scotland, and can recall Christine making the usual Farex, banana, chocolate and milk meals in both Glencoe and Skye. After three days in Skye we all went down with food poisoning, except for Bernard who of course was having most of his food boiled. Eileen and I were sick and felt awful; Christine was sick but did not feel quite so ill, and David was sick but did not feel ill at all. The sickness continued, and David came out in spots reminiscent of chickenpox or measles, so we made a hurried farewell, and went in search of the nearest doctor thirty miles away at Broadford. The doctor was at lunch when we arrived, so we ate our lunch in the car; as we did so, we saw to our surprise, and even to our dismay, that David's spots were slowly vanishing. Thus the doctor was presented with an entirely healthy David, but he politely said food poisoning and prescribed sulphonamide tablets for us all. We then left for the healthier climes of Glen Torridon. This episode was to be the first of a long series of occasions when Bernard has not been ill or affected by upsets when nearly everybody else in the family has gone down. It was a clear indication that Bernard was quite tough, and was not going to drop dead at the first sight of a microbe.

Bernard, aged one

Just after Christmas Christine left us to take up a secretarial post, and her place was filled by Cilli from München. Our first picture of Bernard (*Plate* 2) was taken during our Easter holiday, and shows him sitting up beside Cilli. At that time he could not sit up unaided, and still needed a certain amount of propping with pillows to keep him upright. However, by the time Whit week arrived, he was able to sit upright all by himself, as we see in *Plate* 3. Bernard was now 19 months old, so that by ordinary standards he was making slow progress. As a rough rule of thumb, it seemed that he took twice as long as an ordinary child to reach a particular stage, or even a little longer. We can see that his progress was slow all through this year by looking at *Plate* 5 which shows him a year later when he does not appear greatly changed.

His diet continued much as before, with one important exception. He now agreed to be fed with sausage as well as banana. We were glad of this addition to his intake of protein, and also somewhat curious as to whether he had eaten his first sausage in mistake for the similarly shaped banana. In order to extend his diet further, Eileen began to feed him with sandwiches made from slices of sausage and banana. These sandwiches were cut into small pieces and fed to Bernard a piece at a time. Bernard accepted the sandwiches easily enough, but resolutely refused to accept any filling other than banana or sausage.

During this year Bernard began to show more signs of personality. *Plate 4a* shows him about to let us know that he does not like something. *Plate 4b* is an early shot of what was to be a favourite occupation for many months. Given the least opportunity he would invariably pull at the tablecloth on any table. Therefore it was always necessary to anticipate this move, and place him where he could not reach the cloth.

Another indication that he might not be quite so placid in the months to come appeared when he had to have his hair cut. Taking him to the hairdresser was an extremely difficult business. Although the hairdresser was kind and co-operative, Bernard would not sit still, and yelled most of the time. There was never any question of his hair being cut so that it looked smart: Eileen was only too glad if any hair was cut at all.

Another sign of awakening activity came in May. Hitherto he had always slept quietly and soundly through the night, but now each night he started to cry at about two o'clock, and Eileen had to go down to see him. He usually wanted a drink, or to be tucked in, or a cuddle, or a change of nappies. (Bernard was still wet and dirty. We had made no attempt to train him, as his mental age was still so low that it would have been a complete waste of time to try.) Bernard appeared to like these visits from Mummy, and she came to expect his cries each night at about two o'clock.

Following on the advice mentioned in the previous chapter we were now expecting our third child at about the end of June. Eileen was in very good health until almost the end of the pregnancy. However in May she had to look after Cilli, who was suffering from an infectious form of tonsilitis. Possibly as a result of this, Eileen herself succumbed in June to an extensive infection which was detected in routine tests about three weeks before the expected date of arrival. Eileen was immediately taken into the maternity hospital, where for two days she complained loudly that there was nothing the matter with her. However, her doubts were then put to rest by the arrival of a combination of pneumonia, tonsilitis and nephritis, and she was really quite ill.

Eileen had, of course, been very worried lest there should be something wrong with this new baby. The labour was not quite straightforward, and Eileen recalls watching the doctor prepare for a forceps delivery.

'You will be careful, won't you,' she said.

'Of course,' said the surgeon.

Eileen was not altogether convinced by this conversation, but in the end did not require the help of forceps. As Andrew was delivered, her heart leapt up, for she saw that he was sucking two fingers. She knew by now that this sucking was an indication of some intelligence, just as Bernard's dribbling had been a sign the other way. Andrew was weighed, and turned the scale at a satisfactory 9 lb. He was then passed over for an examination by Keith Lovell, who had come along as soon as he had heard that Andrew was on his way. He was soon able to tell Eileen that Andrew was apparently free from any defects.

Although Andrew was in good health, Eileen had to spend another three weeks in the hospital in isolation, recovering from the various infections. When I was visiting her one day, shortly after Andrew's birth, she said:

'Who is going down to Bernard these nights?'

'What do you mean?' I said.

'Well,' said Eileen. 'When I was at home, he used to cry every night, and I had to go down to him at two o'clock. What's happening now?'

This was rather a sad story. I had always been a sounder sleeper than Eileen, and had seldom heard Eileen getting up to deal with Bernard. The fact of the matter was that neither I nor Cilli had ever heard Bernard cry in the night during all the time that Eileen had been away. Moreover, we had forgotten that Bernard would expect someone to visit him. Almost certainly he must have had an unhappy night or two at first, crying in vain for some attention. However, he must have decided after only a few nights that there was not much future in this activity, for ever afterwards he always slept peacefully through the whole night, except on very rare occasions.

Eileen returned home in the middle of July and her mother came to stay with us. I then left for a conference in the USA. While I was away Cilli went back home, and was replaced by Dorritt. We had been very fortunate with our first two *au-pair* girls, Christine and Cilli, but Dorritt was to show that things were not always so good. She could not cook and was not particularly interested in children, in complete contrast to what she had told us in her letters. Moreover, as her command of the English language was virtually nil, these letters must have been written by a friend. However, she was at least an extra pair of hands, and a baby-sitter.

I returned from the USA at the end of August, and at the end of September we all went for a short holiday in Eskdale, with my mother. Eileen had by then almost completely recovered. She was feeding Andrew herself, and came out with me for walks either in the morning or afternoon. We also recall that Bernard was now able to take his meals with us in the hotel, though of course these still consisted of the inevitable sausage and banana sandwiches cut into small pieces.

Bernard, aged two

During this year Bernard went through the crawling stage, he began to pull himself up in his playpen, and eventually started to walk. We cannot recall that his progress was different in kind from that of David, but each stage lasted longer. He shared the pram with Andrew, who at first was to be seen lying down at one end, with Bernard sitting up at the other. By the time we went on holiday in August, Bernard and Andrew were the same size, Andrew then being $1\frac{1}{4}$ and Bernard $2\frac{1}{2}$ years (*Plate 5*). On this holiday, by some coincidence, Bernard took his first step on the day that Andrew first crawled.

Bernard was still living mainly on sandwiches plus sausage and banana, but we gradually introduced him to a more normal diet. He did not take to this readily. He disliked new tastes, and found the food less easy to eat than sandwiches. His hands were (and still are) small and clumsy. He could not manage a spoon or pusher, and food found its way all too easily from the plate to the table, and then to the floor. As I have already mentioned, he would always grab at a hanging tablecloth, so this luxury was dispensed with.

About this time he learnt his first real word — 'No', or rather 'Nah'. If frustrated at a meal, everything within reach would be pushed across the table so as to make as much mess as possible. (He never threw anything, he just pushed.) If Eileen wanted to

29

say: 'That is not the way to behave', she had first to move everything out of his reach. Then he could only scream. If not at table,
he might sit down and refuse to budge. He would then have to
be carried from place to place, struggling and kicking. Fortunately
we did not know that these habits would continue for another ten
or eleven years. Even at the age of fourteen, he could still revert to
his old habits if in a really cross mood.

Although 'Nah' was now Bernard's favourite word, he
fortunately did not use it the whole time, and some of our pictures
show him as a happy little boy. In fact, on occasion, he was quite
well behaved, particularly if I was present. We certainly had no
hesitation about taking him in the car with the rest of the family
across France to spend our holiday in an apartment in Switzerland.
On the journey we would arrive at an hotel about five o'clock, and
give the children a meal of bread and butter, jam, cheese, biscuits
and milk in their bedroom. Then after a wash they were put to
bed and we had our own meal. In the morning the two youngest
were fed in the bedroom, and then we all came downstairs for
breakfast. During all this travelling Bernard was really as well
behaved as his brothers.

Another aspect of Bernard began to show itself on Saturday
mornings. Saturday was our *au pair* girl's day off, and it was
Eileen's habit to work about the house in the morning, and cook
cakes or buns for the weekend. David had always been happy to
sit and watch these activities, but with Bernard present it was a
very different matter. Any article on the table, a basin or a flour
bin, that Eileen was not holding in both hands, would get pushed
over. At first, she tried to continue her Saturday morning cooking
by putting everything on shelves out of reach, but eventually she
gave up. Baking cakes was not all that important: there was no
point in getting cross and irritated over something that was not
essential. It was much better for Eileen to attempt less so that she
did not feel frustrated.

Once again Bernard was completely different from David. The
normal toddler is always exploring everything, wanting to find out
and learn. A mother helps him to do this; she shows him how things
work, and guides his attention to matters within his capabilities.
By and large, our other children at this stage wanted to please
Eileen rather than make her cross, and it had been a joy to her to
watch them at their discoveries, but with Bernard things were
quite different. There was no attempt at co-operation. He did not

behave like a normal toddler on these occasions until he was about ten. Eileen had to anticipate what Bernard might think of next, to survey the scene of the battlefield, and remove anything that might cause trouble. Any lack of care on her part meant that the cooking, sooner or later, landed on the kitchen floor.

Keith Lovell had warned us that mongols were 'destructive', but that they were also affectionate and lovable. We were certainly beginning to see what Keith meant by destructive, indeed Bernard was such a nuisance at times that it was difficult to view him as an altogether lovable character. That was to come later.

Bernard, aged three

By the summer of this year Andrew was 2 years old and slightly taller than Bernard at 3¾ years. They were the same weight, and were dressed alike. They were both completely mobile and running around, and had learnt how to go safely up and down stairs. On the whole, however, they preferred to be pushed around in the pram, sitting up one at each end. On shopping expeditions the pram was quite essential, so that Bernard and Andrew could be left outside a shop with only the occasional squall and squawk of protest.

This year also saw some improvement on the nappy front. All through 1958 both Bernard and Andrew had been in nappies all the time, being both wet and dirty. This year, however, both of them were dry by day although not at night. Andrew was also clean at night, but not, alas, Bernard.

Plate 6 shows us on our summer holiday in Switzerland. At the end of the holiday Christine's sister, Bärbel, who had been with us for 18 months, returned to Germany. I had to attend a conference at Copenhagen, so Eileen was left to drive home in the car with the children and her mother. As in the previous year, the children had a supper of bread and jam in the hotel bedroom, but everybody went downstairs to take breakfast together in the hotel lounge. All through the journey home Bernard behaved himself well enough to give no particular trouble.

Bernard, aged four

By now Bernard was beginning to look appreciably older and bigger, as is shown in *Plate 7*. He looks very vacant in this shot, but his appearance could vary from day to day, or rather from week to week. For example *Plate 8*, taken a year later, shows him at his best. The difference in appearance in the two pictures is not just due to the camera catching a different fleeting expression on each occasion. At times he looked (and still looks) much more vacant than at others. For reasons which we do not understand at all, but which are probably connected with his metabolism, his level of intelligence appears to go in cycles. For a few weeks he is lively, with an apparently increased intelligence, then this period is followed by a few weeks when his understanding is clearly depressed below its earlier level.

Although he was still very messy at meal times he was slowly starting to improve. In fact, he could now eat reasonably well, but was very reluctant to do so. We say more about his meal-time habits in chapter 9, but must mention here one of his most tiresome tricks, namely that his behaviour was often very much worse when I was not present. For example, when Eileen had prepared a meal for the children, she would call them, saying it was ready. David and Andrew would then come in and sit down, but Bernard would most probably go and sit under the kitchen table. If he happened to be in a good mood he would allow Eileen to coax him from beneath the table, carry him into the dining-room, and sit him on his chair. If he was in a bad mood, he would scream and kick as he was carried to his seat. This was a side of Bernard that I did not see much of, for he behaved very much better when I was at home. Similarly, if I took him out in public he always behaved reasonably well, but if Eileen took him shopping he was quite likely to throw a tantrum and lie down on the floor. We say more about these shopping expeditions in chapter 10.

Even though Bernard was now almost 5 years old, he was only just beginning to play with toys like a normal child. His favourite occupation was knocking down towers of bricks, but he certainly did not want to build them up himself. He would only play if either Eileen or the *au pair* girl were with him, and were prepared to build up the blocks. He resolutely refused to do anything by himself. Even if Eileen or the girl were in the same room he would either just watch them or (more likely) make a thorough nuisance of himself. He made no attempt to play with David and Andrew, even though Andrew was already playing with David. In fact Andrew had played with David as soon as he was able to push a Dinky toy along the floor, but then Bernard was not interested in Dinky toys.

Taking Bernard out shopping proved to be rather a trial for Eileen, but on Saturday afternoons she was able to take all three children on an expedition to the swings about a mile away. Most of the way was by quiet streets or lanes with little or no traffic. Even so, these expeditions were not always uneventful. For example, Andrew might be in the pram, while Bernard and David were walking ahead. Bernard would then decide to do something different, and turn round and walk in the opposite direction. Eileen had then to leave the pram, run to Bernard, pick him up and return him to the pram, and then catch up with David. It would be wrong to give the impression that Bernard was naughty like this *all* the time, but this type of episode certainly occurred very frequently. However, he was still quite small so, unless Eileen was overtired for some reason, she could deal with these situations without getting upset by Bernard's behaviour.

Shortly after Easter Bernard began going to school. Although we had been shown the ESN school, it had always been fairly clear to us that Bernard was only qualified for the lower-grade school, then known as an occupation centre. We therefore never queried the decision that he should start at the occupation centre. Each morning Eileen took him about a mile down the road where a coach picked him up at 9.30, took him to school and brought him back at 3.30. Bernard seemed quite willing and ready to go off in this way, though of course he was quite unable to give us any idea of what went on at the centre.

Chapter 6

Reactions to Bernard

We have already described some of the various problems which arose in dealing with Bernard. However, one of the things which we found most difficult, was to talk about him to others, and to deal with situations where he became involved with other people. Eileen bore the brunt of these difficulties. A mother is expected to talk more about her children than a father, and she is generally more emotionally involved in their progress than he is.

For the first few months after learning that Bernard was a mongol, Eileen could not tell anybody about his condition without becoming emotionally upset. When she went to tell her parish priest, she stood in front of him in tears for several minutes before being able to say anything. When she saw some of her closest friends, who had already heard the news from me, she was hardly in a better state.

We recall going out to tea, quite early on, with some acquaintances. Bernard was left in his pram outside. He did not cry at all, and when we left our hostess said 'What a model baby'. 'Yes', we replied, but could think of nothing else to say. As we pushed him home, Eileen said to me: 'We are having the easiest time now. At present he is flat on his back in the pram, and no one can see him.' Eileen went to some pains to avoid conversations like this. She crossed the road rather than have someone ask after the new baby, and she visited the clinic at two o'clock, a time when no other mothers were likely to be there.

Eileen now went through a long period of acclimatisation. She deliberately tried to avoid thinking about Bernard too much. At first, she particularly tried not to think about the fact that he was a mongol. Later, when he became troublesome, she had to force herself not to dwell on the things which went wrong. After she had put him to bed in the evening, she would try to forget what had gone on during the day. She began each day as if the previous one had not existed. She did not want to tell people about Bernard's naughty deeds, or about the trouble they caused her. She seldom told me of all the things that went amiss.

Looking back, it seems that Eileen was helped at this stage by two circumstances. Every morning she continued with her experiments at the laboratory, where everyone else was busy at their work. It was not a place where one talked about one's children much anyway, and she was able to occupy herself with quite different matters. Our closest friends at the laboratory, who knew all about Bernard, never referred to him, and the others were not really interested in babies. Second, I believed that these very emotional reactions were part of an unhappy transition stage, which we should try to get through as quickly as possible. Eileen knew that I felt strongly on this, and could talk calmly about him if I were present.

We eventually learnt to talk about Bernard as we did about our other children, but it was a slow business spread over several years. Before Bernard was born, Eileen had been in the habit of going to a club for university wives which met in the evening once a week. It was a useful club to which the wives of visiting lecturers could be brought to be introduced to each other and to the locals. It was a friendly gathering and she used to enjoy her occasional women-only evenings. Families were seldom discussed at the club, but after Bernard was born she did not dare venture there in case she should be asked about the new baby. Even when Eileen had grown out of the stage of being upset at the mere mention of Bernard, she still did not go. She was still in the stage of trying not to think about him too much, and so did not want to talk about him. However, as a result of her efforts, she eventually became able to talk normally about Bernard, but it was a long time before she was able to say to a complete stranger that one of her children was a mongol.

As Bernard grew older, he began to sit up in his pram, and so became more noticeable. We particularly recall one day on holiday when Eileen took Bernard and Andrew for an outing in the pram. Bernard was nearly 3 years old and about the same size as Andrew, then 14 months old. During the walk two ladies came towards Eileen; as they approached, Andrew was facing them and Bernard had his back to them. The two ladies beamed at Eileen, and obviously thought that she was the mother of two fine twins. They turned their heads to look at Bernard and their faces fell. The beam turned off and they looked away. Eileen continued, hurt.

Eileen certainly did not enjoy the curious looks and backward glances aimed at Bernard. Even so, they were not as bad as she had feared when first told about Bernard. What she had dreaded proved to be less painful and more bearable than she had thought. Of course, she was helped by having David and Andrew as normal children, and also by the natural acceptance of Bernard by all our friends in Oxford. It was particularly noticeable that the tradespeople, in shops or calling at our house, usually showed a natural acceptance of Bernard. Of course, he did not look *too* conspicuous. Not everybody turned and stared.

As time went on Eileen got more used to taking Bernard about. When he first started school, she had to take him a mile down the road each morning to wait for the coach, but she seldom saw people she knew. Similarly, there were very few people about when she took him to the swings. Acclimatising herself to the situation in this way, she gradually found herself taking Bernard about more and more. However, while Eileen was getting used to Bernard, Bernard was becoming more difficult by attracting attention to himself. Most children pass through a naughty, screaming stage, but Bernard entered this stage at the age of about four and stayed in it until he was about ten.

It is certainly hard if people stare too much at your children's antics, but you have to accept the fact that this is unavoidable. People look at normal children who are being naughty, and stare at anything out of the ordinary. (Bernard himself is the biggest starer of all. If he sees a man with crutches he goes right up to have a good look, and says to him, 'Poor man'.)

Once you realise that you have to accept the stares then it is not too difficult, and you eventually become more or less accustomed to them. The position became easier as the years went by. If Bernard is walking along and behaving himself, people do not generally notice anything unusual about him. However, there is no doubt that his face did attract attention when he was younger, quite probably because he was often seen in the company of his younger and quite normal brother Andrew.

We recently saw a pamphlet about the mentally handicapped, which included the advice : 'You can recognise that mental retardation is a normal occurrence in any community in the world. You can show your acceptance of this by being neither over-curious nor under-interested in the handicapped person and his family.' This is sound advice, but if one pauses for a moment, one sees that there is a very delicate dividing line between being over-curious and under-interested. Not surprisingly, both Eileen and I felt that some reactions to Bernard fell into one or other of these categories. Of course, these categories are not clear cut, because the effect of a remark depends not only on what is said, but also on the state of mind of the parents. Yet at times we could clearly distinguish both under-interest and over-curiosity, and genuine interest. It is easiest to illustrate what we mean by some examples.

The under-interested were small in number, but clearly recognisable. When Bernard was about a year old, Eileen met an acquaintance whom she knew quite well. Mrs A asked Eileen how we all were, and Eileen asked after her family. She said she had had another child, and Eileen said 'So have we'. Then as Mrs A was a doctor, Eileen thought it was safe to add 'He's a mongol'. 'Oh, is he?' she said. 'Well, must go, goodbye.' Perhaps she was embarrassed, but Eileen was left with the feeling of having made some social gaffe.

As another example, Eileen wrote to a long-standing friend telling her about Bernard. The friend then wrote to other friends of Eileen's, passing on the news, and telling them not to write to Eileen at all. She herself has not been near Eileen since, but telephoned Eileen's mother some years later and asked: 'Have they still got the funny little boy?' 'Of course', said Granny rather sharply and crossly.

Although the term under-interested describes a very recognisable state of mind, over-curious covers a much wider spectrum of reactions. Some people give the impression that they are mainly interested in knowing how difficult things are for the mother. They do not show much concern for the child, but wish to learn about the dreadful state the family must be in. They relish horror stories, and make a point of asking for details which you would prefer not to give. Above all, they don't appear to enjoy the fact that you are coping with the situation. Instead, they tell you of all the families where the child has had to be placed in an institution, a hospital or a home.

Another version of being over-curious takes the form of what Eileen calls the pressure group. For an example, we heard of the case of a mother who had previously looked after her grown-up mongol sister at home, together with her young family. This mother had then decided (we are sure quite rightly) that it was bad for the children to be brought up in a home dominated by an elderly mongol. She had therefore arranged for her sister to live in a local institution, where she was visited regularly, taken out, and was apparently quite happy. However, we were told that because the mother had put her sister into a home, she thought that everyone else should do the same.

As the years have gone by, Eileen has learnt that she herself can sometimes encourage a form of over-curiosity. There is now an increasing amount of genuine interest in and awareness of the problems of mentally handicapped children. Yet people do not meet many families with such children. When they realise that Eileen is prepared to talk about Bernard they begin to ask questions and show an interest. There is a lot to tell them, but one must avoid the danger of talking solely about Bernard.

Genuine interest is again hard to define but very easy to recognise. Our mothers could not have been kinder or more sympathetic. Eileen's brother and sister-in-law have always treated Bernard just like our other children. We were fortunate in our own friends. Not long after Bernard was born, Eileen was visited unexpectedly by a friend she had not seen for some time. Diana had known that we were expecting a baby, so Eileen had to tell her all about Bernard. Diana said something like 'Oh, the lamb', and picked him up and cuddled him. She was about the first person who really did cuddle him. Eileen suddenly realised that sometimes he had been treated kindly enough, but rather as a curiosity.

I have mentioned that we first took Bernard to Chapel Farm in the Lake District when he was 6 months old, and he has been there every year since. Everyone on the farm accepts Bernard as he is, and they have always treated him as they treat all our other children. Perhaps that is not quite true; they do spoil him a little, but then Mrs Weir spoils all the children. The Weirs could not have been kinder. Their complete acceptance of Bernard as he was, and as he is, has been most comforting to us all. Mrs Weir has never asked an awkward question, yet she always enquires about his progress and schooling, and is as pleased as we are when there is some progress to report.

Bernard is particularly attached to Mrs Weir's sons. They have taken him everywhere, on the milk-run, around the fields repairing walls, into the kitchen at breakfast, and they have even taught him how to milk a cow. They have played with him and teased him. They have sat him on top of the cows, and brought him down when he screamed. But then all the children have been up on top of the cows at one time or another, and Bernard would have felt dreadfully out of it if he had not been put on top himself.

Many people, however, find a very real difficulty in knowing how best to respond to the unusual situations associated with mental handicap. The reactions of our two mothers to Bernard were a case in point. Eileen's mother had a friend with a grown-up mongol daughter, Nina, whom we mentioned in chapter 2. The arrival of Bernard was therefore not an entirely new situation, but one which she knew how to deal with. She always managed to say the right thing. My mother was equally, or even more sympathetic, but at first tended to make rather too much of our problems.

Some people, of course, know nothing of mental handicap. When Bernard was 10 months old, we spent a few days in an hotel in Scotland. David had his meals with us in the dining-room, but Bernard was fed in our bedroom, after Christine had prepared his food in the hotel kitchen. This was the period when we took some delightful photographs of David, but none of Bernard. During the visit one member of the kitchen staff asked Christine: 'How is it that Mr and Mrs Wilks have a Chinese baby?'

At the other end of the spectrum one always finds it easy to talk naturally to parents who themselves have a child who is handicapped in some way. On the same holiday in Scotland we stayed for a week or so in a house where there was a little girl aged about three, with a stunted foot and deformed fingers. Looking back she seems to have been a forerunner of the thalidomide children. She was a pretty little girl who could run about and use her hands perfectly well, but her mother was very upset at her disfigurement. She and Eileen talked together, and she was apparently consoled at the sight of Bernard. She now seemed grateful that her child was not as badly off as ours.

On another holiday, we spent the night at a small hotel in France near the Jura. At the time Bernard was about 10 years old. As we were leaving in the morning Madame asked kindly: 'How old is your little son?' This was an unusual question, so we were not surprised to learn that she had a son like Bernard, of about the same age. 'He does not live with us you understand: in an establishment like this it would not be possible. He is in a home not very far from here.' We gained the impression that she was sorry that the little boy was not at home with her.

Just as people find it difficult to talk to parents, so they find it difficult to behave naturally with handicapped children. Many people speak to them quite differently from the way they do to normal children. For example, when Eileen was out with Bernard, and perhaps Andrew or David, someone might say to Bernard: 'Hello, young fellow', and pat him on the head. Bernard would look at him blankly, as if he were thinking: 'Who the heck are you?' No stranger ever patted and addressed David and Andrew in this way. Bernard found their attitude strange, and was obviously not too happy about it.

People were often much more friendly to Bernard than to a normal child. They would joke with him, tease him, and slap him on the back. The effect on Bernard was disastrous, for he would become over-excited and cheeky, and very soon objectionable and troublesome. Then Eileen had the utmost difficulty in getting him out of the resulting situation. Of course, normal children can behave in this way, but never with the frequency and persistence shown by Bernard.

Even though some people seem to bring out the worst in Bernard, others instinctively bring out the best. Eileen recalls a party after David's confirmation, when Bernard was about 8 years old. Bernard had been well behaved all through the confirmation. He had been at the front of the church so that he could see the whole service without anyone being in his way, and he had been quiet and inconspicuous. At the party afterwards, it was obvious that he was relaxing his restraint a little, and Eileen wondered how long 'he would last'. At that moment, one of the priests went up to her to say hello, and it became clear that Bernard was getting rather edgy.

'I'll just ignore him,' he said. 'I think that's the best thing to do.'

'How right you are,' Eileen murmured gratefully, as she watched Bernard subside beside them into a quiet little boy.

One day when Eileen had taken the children to a service at Blackfriars, the Dominican church in Oxford, Bernard began to fidget and was quite obviously preparing to stage a strike. Eileen began to fear a loud and audible 'Nah' and was trying to control him quietly, when all of a sudden he subsided. She saw that one of the Dominican priests in the choir was scowling fiercely at him. She smiled gratefully back at the priest, and all was peaceful. It really was quite amusing how Bernard had been reduced to silence by just one scowl at the right moment. The Dominicans have been particularly successful in accepting Bernard as he is. They treat him no differently from our other children, and have always shown a sympathetic understanding of the problems he presents.

Chapter 7

In the USA

In 1960 I was invited to spend the second half of the year as a visiting professor at Yale University, in New Haven, Connecticut, so we all went to live in the USA for six months. At the time David was six, Andrew three and Bernard five, and a new brother or sister was clearly on the way. In addition, we were accompanied by Eileen's 17-year-old niece, Anne, to help look after the children.

This visit to the USA presented us with a kaleidoscopic array of glittering impressions. The cold, the heat, the humidity, and the deep crystal blue of the clear winter sky. Like nearly everyone before us, we were impressed by the zest and enthusiasm in American life, by the tremendous range of views and outlooks one encountered journeying about the country, and in particular by the kindness and hospitality of our American hosts. We also find it particularly easy to recall Bernard as he was then. Looking back over the years, it is not always easy to remember when Bernard first did this or that, or what he was like at any particular time. However, some days and events remain in the memory because of unusual or out of the ordinary circumstances. Our visit to the USA acts as one such reference point and makes it possible to recall several impressions of Bernard as he was then.

Although Bernard could at times be very tiresome about the house, he was sufficiently well behaved on the *Mauretania* for us all to have a very pleasant voyage to New York. He shared a bunk with Andrew, and took to life on board ship without any upset or disturbance, but with considerable curiosity. Like his two brothers, he was overawed by the size and decor of the restaurant, and was on his best behaviour from the beginning. He was then able to use a spoon as a fork, and really behaved himself very well. Between meals, he spent quite a lot of time with his brothers in the nursery, playing with other children under the eye of a trained attendant. When we left them on the first morning there were some indignant and persistent cries, but hard-heartedly we took no notice. The cries diminished and then ceased, and when we looked in the nursery an hour later we saw all three, playing happily among the toys, together with some other children. From then on they returned to the nursery each day, became very friendly with the girl in charge, and thoroughly enjoyed themselves.

Perhaps the chief highlight of the voyage for Bernard was watching the bell-boy, one of whose jobs was to summon people to meals by walking round the ship striking his call bells. The bell-boy was also the lift-boy, and Bernard's other main joy was going up and down in the lifts. Eileen had an anxious moment one day when she went to collect him from the nursery and was told that he had already left with Anne. Having just seen Anne, Eileen knew this to be incorrect. We started to look for him. It was quite a time before the nursery attendant remembered that it was not Anne who had collected him but the bell-boy. So we started to trail the lift. When we eventually found ourselves on the same floor as the lift, there was Bernard, happy as a sandboy, going up and down. He was less happy at being removed.

We still remember disembarking from the *Mauretania*, partly because of our experience just as we were going aboard at Southampton. The passport official, instead of flicking through Eileen's passport, as he had flicked through mine, turned the pages slowly and carefully, and then remarked that it was not valid for the USA! It had a current American visa, but was an old passport in which the countries to which Eileen could go were specifically listed, and the USA was not on the list. At this late hour, there was nothing to do but hope that no one would notice the omission. When we arrived in New York, we were all seen by the immigration officials in one of the ship's lounges. Eileen sat with the children, while I stood in a queue with all our passports. At the same time various officials were strolling around, including a pleasant-looking man in an olive green uniform. Eventually he made his way towards Eileen and the children, and told her that he was from the health department. He remarked that he had noticed Bernard, and asked how he was, how Eileen managed with him, how long we were coming for, what I did, where we were from, did Bernard go to school, and how healthy he was. The official was friendly, and Eileen had a pleasant enough chat with him, even though she was all the time anxiously watching my progress up the queue with her passport. Fortunately, no one noticed anything wrong with this document, and we left the ship without difficulty. It was only afterwards that we began to wonder whether the pleasant official in the olive green uniform could have refused us entry on account of Bernard!

For our first few weeks in New Haven we lived in a delightful old house with a fine large garden. We had only been there a few days when we found that Bernard had learnt how to open a gate. Eileen suddenly noticed that he was no longer in the garden, and rushed off to look for him. Although he had not been long gone, he was already across the road, and in a park on the other side. Henceforth, the garden gate had to be carefully locked, and an eye kept on Bernard, as he was only too willing to repeat this performance. Soon after our arrival we had the good fortune to spend a fortnight in a country cottage in the White Mountains at Randolph, New Hampshire. This comfortable wooden house stood by itself in a wide clearing in the thick forest that covers so much of New England. When we arrived, we were rather disconcerted to see that the clearing, which also served as the garden, was not fenced off in any way from the wood. After our recent experience in New Haven, we had visions of Bernard and his two brothers wandering off into the woods, and never being seen again. However, we need not have worried, for the woods and their undergrowth turned out to be so thick that none of the children could penetrate it for more than a foot or so.

When we returned to New Haven, it was still very hot, so Eileen sometimes took the children to the nearest good beach by the sea. This was at Hamanasett, some thirty miles away, but quite near by American standards, with the help of the Connecticut turnpike. On their first visit, the beach was very crowded, but they found a place for Andrew and Bernard to paddle, while Anne started to teach David to swim. Bernard soon tired of paddling and making sand castles, and was attracted to other families on their own small patches of sand, particularly if they were having tea or ice cream. He would continually wander off to stand and stare. In the end Eileen had no choice but to cut short her rest by the sea, and take him for a walk to a less attractive part of the beach, where there were more rocks and brambles but fewer people. When they returned home they reported to me that they were the only party on the beach that had actually gone swimming. However, this pride in English achievement only lasted a short while, for we saw in the evening paper that on the previous day a swimmer on the coast of New Jersey, not far away, had been attacked by a shark!

At the beginning of September we moved into the house where we were to live for most of our stay. This was in the township of Hamden, situated about five miles north of New Haven, essentially a dormitory area for the city. By and large, we did not see a great deal of the people living around us, although Eileen met several people at church, and some of the mothers of David's friends. One of our next-door neighbours was waiting to greet us as we drove up to our house for the first time, but we soon found that her principal concern was to tell us that the slantwise boundary between the two houses precluded us from taking our car into our drive. We did not get around to discussing Bernard very much. However, the reactions of most people were not unlike those at home, and we did not notice much difference between taking Bernard round in the USA and in England.

As Bernard had already started attending the training school in Oxford, one of our first enquiries was whether he could attend a similar school at New Haven. Our next-door neighbour at our first house was a valuable and friendly source of information on this and other topics. We learned that there was no training centre for mentally handicapped children in New Haven comparable with the state supported school in Oxford. There was a small private school, to which Bernard eventually went, but the state of Connecticut gave no official recognition to the possibility that mentally handicapped children could be cared for at home and attend training centres. There seemed to be no official acceptance that such children could be trained, and we gathered that they were nearly all in institutions of one sort or another. One does not see many mentally retarded children about in England, but we saw not a single other such child during our stay in the USA except at this private school.

The school was run by a few dedicated enthusiasts who felt that something could and should be done for the children. One of these ladies had a handicapped child herself, while another had a grandson who was a mongol. The school was located in the basement of a church hall near the centre of New Haven, provided by the vicar at a nominal rent. The teachers were the two enthusiasts themselves, together with one or two other helpers. We had the

45

curious feeling that we were seeing the way in which the Mabel Prichard school in Oxford had grown up some fifty years earlier.

As the school was such a small venture, Bernard had to pass an entrance examination, or rather he had to be interviewed to see whether he was suitable for the school. This we could well understand. Without a full complement of trained staff, a rough and troublesome child will soon break up a group of other children who are prepared to be co-operative. Bernard did not behave very well at his interview, although not particularly badly. Eileen and Bernard sat down to talk, but one minute later Eileen was up and out of the room to retrieve Bernard who was on his way down the stairs. For the rest of the interview, someone had to take it in turns to guard the door and distract Bernard from doing anything too mischievous, but in the end they accepted him.

Each morning Bernard was collected by taxi at about 9 o'clock and returned home by 1 o'clock as there were no facilities for providing meals at the school. The taxi came directly to our house, and the driver knocked on the door and collected Bernard. Although we had to pay for the taxi, we found this system a tremendous improvement on the drill at home when Eileen often had to wait twice a day on a cold wet street corner for a coach which was often late. Once he arrived at the school, Bernard's activities were not really very much different from those at Oxford. For retarded children as young as he was, the activities in both cases were essentially supervised playgroups. The older children made simple mats, kettle-holders, dolls, knitted squares and such like, in sufficient quantity to be able to hold a sale of work just before Christmas.

We were not in the USA long enough to obtain a very clear picture of American methods of treating and helping the mentally handicapped. However, it seemed that there was a considerable difference in the American and British approach to the provision of day schools, which children could attend while living at home. Because of the lack of these facilities in New Haven, it seemed that some parents might be forced to put their child into an institution, even though they would prefer not to, and even though the child could be usefully trained in a special school. In fact, during our visit we heard that the state of Connecticut had recognised the work being done at the school, and had agreed to help financially, but we left before the details were finally settled. Many people we met assured us that Connecticut was one of the best states in the USA for the treatment of the mentally handicapped. One woman even said that they had moved into Connecticut from another state so that their daughter would be better cared for.

About two weeks before Maureen was born, Eileen and I made a short trip to see Washington. We drove both ways and spent two nights away from home. Rather than leave Anne alone with three boys, we made arrangements for Bernard to stay with a negro family who were used to doing this sort of baby-sitting. We took Bernard to see them before making the final arrangements, they were friendly, there were other children, and there was television. We might have been worried that Bernard would be puzzled by their different colour, but one of our most dependable friends in Oxford is a Jamaican who has cared for all our children in emergencies since they were small. In any case small children generally seem to be unaware of colour differences. On the day we left we took Bernard along, he was welcomed into the television room, kissed us goodbye, and then settled down in front of the television without a moment's hesitation.

On our return from Washington we went to collect Bernard, and immediately realised that something had not been a success. His host said that he had been as good as gold the whole time; he had eaten all his meals, played with the other children, gone for walks, watched the television, and slept well. This was a story which we were to hear several times more in the future when Bernard went away by himself on school holidays. It seemed that while we had been away he was quite happy, but that on our return he suddenly realised that he had been left by himself. He slunk to Eileen and hid his face against her, and clung to her all the way home. It was then about three or four days before he was back to his normal self.

One Saturday, towards the end of September, the weather was so pleasant that we all went off in the afternoon to the Sleeping Giant State Park at the north end of Hamden. This park is a wooded reserve, with small rocky hills running up a few hundred feet to a look-out tower giving a fine view of the rolling forest-land of Connecticut. We decided we would all walk up the hill, as it was not very high; there was a good path, and the top was not much more than a mile away. We started up through the woods, which were quite delightful, the trees rustled, the birds sang, the sun shone fitfully through the leafy glades, and all was at peace, but not for long. Bernard soon decided that he did not think much of the expedition and said so in no uncertain terms. We walked along with Anne and I each holding one of his hands. He was encouraged, he was scolded, he was shouted at, but his only comment was 'Naw, naw, naw, naw', which we translated as repeated requests for 'No more'.

We did not take these protests too seriously, at least at first. We knew that he was a lazy little fellow who would not walk two steps if he could persuade his Mum to push him in the pram or drive him in the car. We also knew that he was 5 years old, healthy and sturdy, and that there was nothing wrong with his legs. When the going became steeper, his squawks produced a side effect on Andrew, and he too started to protest, not quite as loudly as Bernard but very audibly. It thus came about that the Wilks party was spread over a long length of the path. In front David was steaming ahead happily, quite out of sight. Then came Eileen, almost nine months pregnant and ready for a quiet walk, but having to tell Andrew at each turn of the path that we were nearly at the top. Finally, from a long way down the hill could be heard fainter squawks from one of the last three members of the party. However, we all eventually reached the summit. The descent was made much more expeditiously, as none of the children had been made to do anything beyond their powers, and we all saw that the walk had really been quite short. Bernard trotted down back to the car quite happily, and only Eileen was tired by the expedition.

The sequel to our walk up Sleeping Giant followed swiftly, for Maureen was born safely at the Grace New Haven hospital the following morning. Five days later, after paying the hospital charges, I traded my receipt with the ward sister in exchange for Eileen and our new daughter. We then drove home, where everyone was very pleased to greet their little sister. Bernard in particular was very thrilled.

We were, of course, conscious of the need to make sure that Bernard did not do anything silly to the new baby. When Andrew was born, Bernard was not mobile, so there had been no problem in protecting Andrew from Bernard. Then Andrew had grown at such a rate that by the time Bernard was mobile, Andrew was big enough to look after himself. In fact, as far as we could see, Bernard was never aggressive towards Andrew, and we never had cause for worry in bringing the two of them up together. Maureen presented a different situation. We now had a mobile 5-year-old and a tiny baby. We did not risk anything, and Bernard was never left alone with Maureen when she was small. Yet I do not think that we need have worried, for he was never rough with her. He did not want to

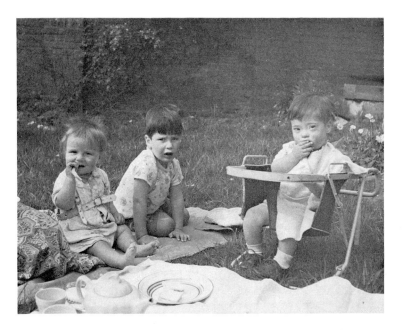

5 Meal-time habits at the age of 2½ years. Bernard does not look very different from his appearance a year ago (*Plate 4*), but is now feeding himself with cut sandwiches. David is 4 years old and Andrew 12 months

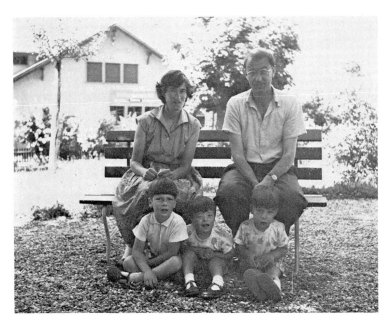

6 A family group taken when David was 5, Bernard 3¾, and Andrew 2

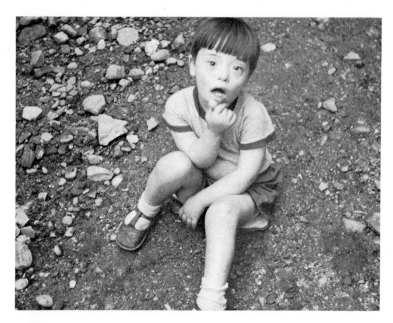

7 A very vacant shot taken at the age of $4\frac{1}{2}$. It is interesting to compare this with *Plate 8* an equally typical shot taken about a year later

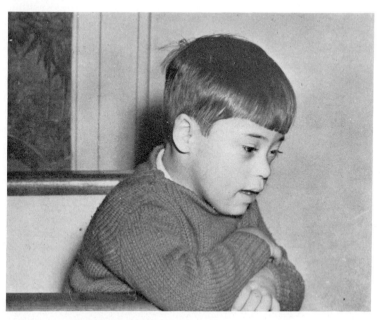

8 On the way home from America, aged 5

pull at her, or push her, or do anything silly or thoughtless that would be dangerous. In fact, we did not need to take any precautions against Bernard that we did not also take against Andrew, who was then only three.

Eileen has always had strong views on the need to avoid arousing jealousies in a family. She had always tried to give the minimum necessary attention to a baby, and the maximum attention to the others. She used to feed Andrew with David and Bernard sitting on her lap, and she fed Maureen with Andrew and Bernard on her lap, with David often beside her. When feeding was over, she would put Maureen down in her cot, tuck her in, and then turn her attention to the others. This policy paid off. Maureen slept, ate and thrived, and the boys did not show any jealousy either then or later. To quote Eileen, 'It's a bit of a do feeding a baby with the others on your lap, but it was fun and it didn't last for long.'

During our visit, Bernard became a television addict. Our first house, like our home in Oxford, had no set, but there was one in our Hamden home. It was rather an old set so we were forced to rely mainly on the local programmes which were often not very good. On the other hand, some of the main network programmes which were relayed were absolutely first class, including the Kennedy-Nixon election debates. The children mainly watched about tea-time, when a large part of the programme was given over to shots of a large dance hall holding jive sessions of young teenagers mooning about on the floor. This, nevertheless, produced a hypnotic effect which held the children's attention.

The viewing was not uninterrupted. Bernard was not content to sit near to the set; he would stand up and get as close to it as possible. He liked to put his face against the screen; we have no idea what he saw, but this was his favourite position. If David and Andrew wanted to see anything, they had to drag him away every few minutes. They also had to contend with his intense interest in anything mechanical which now began to show itself for the first time. He was an inveterate fiddler with all the various control knobs on the front of the set. I think he knew that the knobs would improve the quality of the picture, so he fiddled with them and promptly lost the picture. Sometimes every knob would be turned round as far as it would go. He always got upset when he lost the picture, but during the whole of our stay at Hamden he never learnt that the picture would disappear if he began to fiddle.

Our visit came to an end with the end of the year, and we sailed for home on the *Queen Elizabeth*. Our last night in the USA, spent at an hotel in New York, happened to give us a reference mark on Bernard's power of speech. By now Bernard was trying to talk, but was doing little more than making curious noises. He only had one clear word, 'Naw', which was used to mean either 'No' or 'No more'. When we arrived at the hotel, Bernard and Andrew were put to bed and left to go to sleep. A little later, when we were in our own room, we heard a knock at the door. It was the manager of the hotel, and he was concerned and anxious. The telephonist at the switchboard had been rung up and all she could hear were the most awful grunts and groans. 'Oh,' we said, 'that's Bernard.' Yet when we walked into his room, the telephone was back on its rest and all was peace and quiet!

The voyage home was not much different from our outward journey except there were fewer people on board. During our first meal, Eileen and I had our doubts as to how everyone was going to behave. On the outward journey the children had been somewhat overawed by the restaurant, but it was obvious that their reaction on the *Queen Elizabeth* was: 'Ah, here we are again, now for a nice time.' Fortunately they did not overstep the mark, the passage took only five days, and everyone enjoyed themselves.

Chapter 8

Life with a Mongol Brother

From the beginning it was fairly clear to us that a mongol could make life difficult for his brothers and sisters. If we had had any doubts on this point, they were certainly removed by the number of times we were advised not to let the other children suffer. However, to begin with, there was not much we could do, but wait to see how things turned out.

Because David was our first child he had received Eileen's undivided attention until he was 15 months old. Even before we knew that there was something wrong with Bernard, Eileen took particular care that he still received his fair share of her time. She would leave Bernard asleep in the cot most of the time, and play with David without interruption. As we have mentioned, Bernard took a long time to grow out of the very dormant baby stage. It was a year before he played with a rattle, and almost two years before he started to crawl.

Because Bernard grew up so slowly, David received the same amount of attention as before, and continued to live very much as if he were an only child. Thus one of the first results of Bernard's backwardness was that David did not have a companion with whom he could play. However, when he was 2¼ years old, he began going to a nursery school a quarter of a mile away. He went there every morning and played happily with the other children. At home, David was becoming very much the elder brother, fetching and carrying things for Eileen. He was always helpful and understanding by nature, and as he grew older we never had any difficulty in explaining to him that Bernard was rather on the slow side.

The arrival of Andrew did not affect this picture very much at first. David was then three. He soon became fond of Andrew, but we were careful to see that he was not left alone with him. An inquisitive finger pushed in the wrong place might have dire consequences, and it was better to be safe than sorry. There was no need to take any precautions against Bernard, for he was still unable to get out of his pram or cot.

Our relatively ordered arrangements suffered a severe set-back when Bernard began to crawl. We have already mentioned his delight in knocking things down, and we soon found what we were in for. He liked to knock down columns of bricks. He scattered toys right, left, and centre. As soon as he found a building of bricks, he pushed it over. Andrew was still only about 6 months old, so he was not immediately affected, but David was. Fortunately, none of us realised that Bernard would not begin to grow out of these habits for another ten years!

It was now necessary to separate David from Bernard whenever he wanted to play with his cars, bricks, and other toys. We arranged this separation by Eileen or the *au pair* feeding and bathing Bernard and Andrew together, while the other would play with David. Our foreign girl was thus a very important part of our arrangements, a second pair of hands in the house. Ever since Christine had taken David out for an afternoon walk, we had arranged for her to be employed as a mother's help on a labour permit rather than as an *au pair*. She worked in the morning like an *au pair*, and had time off in the afternoon, but worked again from 3 until 6 o'clock. She had every evening free from about 6 o'clock apart from occasional baby-sitting, and also $1\frac{1}{2}$ days off each week.

Nine months later when Bernard had just arrived at the walking stage, Andrew began to crawl, so they both knocked down David's bricks. David, then coming up to five, went through a very trying period when everything he built had a good chance of being pushed over. He took it all very much as elder brother to the babies, and never lost his temper. A favourite game that amused everybody at this time was for David to build up a pile of bricks, while Eileen would hold back Andrew and a fussing and squawking Bernard. Then Bernard or Andrew were allowed to take it in turns to demolish the whole lot. This was great fun.

A few weeks later, Andrew started to build with the bricks, and then objected strongly to his own work being demolished. He did not mind attacking David's bricks, but Bernard's onslaughts on his own work were quite another matter. Andrew was far more of a builder than David, and enjoyed laying out elaborate constructions, but if Bernard managed to get into the nursery everything would be 'knocked for six' in a matter of seconds. The way in which Bernard could sniff out something to knock down, and the speed with which he could get into the nursery, were just unbelievable. Fortunately Bernard usually confined his efforts to pushing things over rather than throwing them about. Therefore there was never much danger of his doing any damage to Andrew. In any case Andrew was soon the bigger child, and able to look after himself.

From now on we had to keep Bernard away from both David and Andrew when they were playing. On most days, I was seldom home before bedtime, so Eileen would play with David and Andrew or prepare supper, and the girl would play with Bernard in another room. On other days, Eileen would look after Bernard, while the girl would play with David and Andrew. In either case, the extra pair of hands was essential for the play and development of the normal children. This segregation became even more important when David and Andrew began to read. It was only possible for Eileen to read to them, and they to her, if Bernard was kept happily occupied in another room.

The great assistance provided by Christine and her successors was never more obvious than on their afternoon or day off. Eileen would be together with the three children, and at some stage would give her attention to David and Andrew. At this point, Bernard immediately became annoyed: he screamed, he yelled, he knocked bricks over. When it was time for tea he would not budge, and Eileen had to carry him from the nursery to the tea table. It was almost impossible to do anything constructive with David and Andrew when Bernard was in the same room, and Bernard objected to being left alone. He realised that his brothers were getting attention, he wanted attention too, and he objected most strenuously. The only way to obtain peace was for everyone to play at Bernard's level, and for a couple of days a week this had to be accepted.

On most Sunday afternoons Eileen and I would go for a walk by ourselves. Eileen argued that the girl had her day off from Bernard on the Saturday, while she had hers on the Sunday. The girl would take David, Andrew and Bernard to the swings in a nearby park, play there, come home for tea, and put them to bed. She hardly ever found Bernard as troublesome as Eileen did. We never came home to find her as tired and exhausted as Eileen sometimes was after a day alone with the three of them. It seemed that what Bernard particularly resented was his *mother* giving attention to David and Andrew.

As time went on, David and Andrew began to play together, and could be left by themselves. Their activities became more involved and grown-up, but all the time Bernard was hovering in the background ready to play his part. He would take the rubber tyres off their model Dinky cars, and throw them away; fortunately this did not worry the boys as cars can go without rubber wheels. As they grew older, they played football in the garden and Bernard found that he was not able to take a real part in the game. Periodically the football went missing, and we soon learnt that we had to look for it on the other side of the garden wall! When they were older still, David and Andrew started to play chess, a game which held their attention completely, but left no role for Bernard. After a time the chessmen vanished!

It was always necessary for us to be on the watch so that Bernard did not become too great a nuisance to his brothers. When David was about 7 years old, we adopted the stratagem of dividing the nursery into two. This room was large and bare with a plain wooden floor, and contained a stove, an old settee, cupboards for toys, and Bernard's cot and pram. It was not elegant, but there was plenty of space for the boys to run around in, and we did not have to worry about the furniture getting damaged. By arranging the cupboards and chests of drawers in a line across the middle of the room, plus a little home carpentry, we divided the nursery into two halves. The inner half served as a sanctum for David and Andrew where they could leave their model trains and similar toys free from interference by Bernard. All they had to do was to remember to latch the door, which was so arranged that Bernard could not open it. Bernard took a very poor view of these arrangements, and was always on hand ready to rush in and wreak havoc whenever the door was left open by mistake. Fortunately this did not happen too often.

Obviously, David and Andrew, and later Maureen, were well aware of Bernard's presence. What did they think of him? It was clear, at least, that they each looked at him in a rather different light. David had always understood that Bernard was different from other children, and had always looked after him. Eileen recalls that one day, when David was about six, she was out shopping and had left David and Bernard outside the shop together with Andrew in the pram. She looked out to see David having a fight with an unknown little boy, and went out to find what it was all about. David explained: 'He said rude things about Bernard, so I hit him.'

David and Bernard have always been very fond of each other. To Bernard, David has been his great big elder brother. David, for his part, has always been ready to help Bernard, and on occasion to take his part against hard-hearted mum and dad. Since he was about five, he has been a great help to Eileen in keeping Bernard under control, for example on shopping expeditions. Today he is quite prepared to take Bernard for a shopping expedition into the centre of Oxford.

Perhaps as a result of Bernard, the children have tended to play more in their friends' homes than in ours. However, Bernard has kept out of the way of David's and Andrew's friends, behaving like any other younger brother who would not expect to play with a much older brother. We must also remember that Bernard is very small, even today he is not much larger than a 12-year-old. Therefore visitors to the house have not always realised just how backward he is.

Andrew was quite different from David. He was less interested in people, and from an early age was happy to play by himself. His play was at times quite imaginative, and he was obviously a much more self-centred child than David. He was slow to talk, showed no desire to speak, and said little more than one or two words until he was about five. Nevertheless he obtained all he wanted without talking. He was an excellent mime, and confused the experts by being able to read before being willing to talk.

Andrew, being Andrew, did not really understand that there was anything wrong with Bernard until he was about seven. Yet Bernard must have been in some ways a bit of a mystery to him. He was obviously very different from David; in particular he did not talk but made a few odd noises. On the other hand, we suspect that Andrew was not terribly interested in these differences. In any case, he never talked about them until he was seven, and began to bring friends to the house.

When Andrew first went to the nursery school, he was not a companionable little boy, and very seldom had friends to tea. He became more sociable when he moved on to his next school, and would then invite friends home. At this time, everybody might be sitting round the tea-table, when Andrew would point at Bernard and say 'How old do you think he is?' The only persons embarrassed by this question were Eileen and myself. His friends would look blank and say nothing. Andrew would continue: 'Well, he's older than me, he's nine, and he's much smaller than me. And he can't talk either.' Eileen would then stand up for Bernard, and say that Andrew wasn't all that wonderful at talking either. Eventually we had to put an end to these conversations, and told Andrew that he was not to make these remarks to his friends without explaining that Bernard was not quite normal, and moreover that he was not to do this in front of Bernard.

Mentally handicapped children are still sufficiently uncommon that there is some problem in introducing them to strangers. As far as grown-ups are concerned, we just say 'This is Bernard', and trust that our visitor will be able to see for himself that Bernard is somewhat different. With children, however, matters are more difficult. They probably have no knowledge of mental handicap, and certainly not of mongolism, and one cannot explain all this to them in front of Bernard, who has a fairly good idea of what people are saying about him. Once, for example, the children met several other children playing around the fields and farmyard at Chapel Farm. According to Maureen, these children saw Bernard as a little Chinese boy whom they could not understand, and who was very small for his age. They just did not know what was wrong. They did not play with him, but then Bernard did not want to play with them.

Maureen's attitude to Bernard has been characteristically different from that of both her brothers. To David, Bernard has always been a younger and smaller brother. To Andrew, he must have seemed a rather mysterious kind of twin, but to Maureen he was for quite a time just another elder brother. His behaviour may have seemed a little odd at times, but then big brothers tend to be a law unto themselves. However, Maureen was much more matter-of-fact and percipient of everyday details than Andrew. By the time she was five, she had realised that Bernard was quite different from his brothers, and we had been able to explain to her that Bernard was backward and would remain so.

When Maureen was two she went, like David and Andrew, to the nursery school, where she played with children of her own age. In a year or two, however, she found that she had an excellent playmate in Bernard. She was ready to arrange his play and tell Bernard what to do, and Bernard was always ready to accept her orders. At times it seemed to us as if she had a great big glorious doll. Be that as it may, they certainly got on very well together. As far as we can tell, she has accepted him completely.

Today, we have the impression that David, Andrew and Maureen have suffered no great harm by growing up with a mongol brother. However, when Bernard was born, it seemed that he might present a very serious problem. We talked to friends who themselves had been seriously embarrassed by backward brothers or sisters, and we learnt of families whose life was distorted to a remarkable extent by the presence of a backward child. It was clear to us that a mentally handicapped child could be a source of trouble and unhappiness to his brothers and sisters. We had to face the question of how much disruption of their own lives we should expect our children to bear on Bernard's behalf. We decided that we would not ask our other children to do anything for Bernard which they were not really willing to do.

From the start, I felt that as Bernard grew up, he might become very difficult and unsociable. It was therefore a possibility that it might eventually be best to place him in an institution. However, when we first learned that Bernard was a mongol, there was clearly no need to take any immediate action. We were able to take our time in thinking what special arrangements we should make for him. There was no particular hurry.

When Bernard was about two, I made a determined attempt to get Eileen to agree, not that Bernard should go into a home, but that there was a possibility that it *might* be necessary in the future. I was anxious that this problem should be faced, and that a decision should not come about merely by accepting the status quo. Eileen found this question unpalatable; to talk of putting her very own baby, albeit a mongol, into an institution was most unwelcome. She went to seek advice from one of the parish priests. To her dismay, he talked of the possible harm that could come to the mother if she identified herself too closely with the handicapped child. He pointed out that the children's friends might react against Bernard, and finally stressed that in dealing with Bernard we must not put ourselves in his place. Eileen then went to consult Dr Stewart. He saw that she was very upset and worried, and pointed out that in any case nothing need be done immediately. We both agreed, Eileen because she did not want Bernard to go away at all, and I because there was no need at the moment.

As Bernard grew up during the next five years, it became

apparent that he placed considerable strain on the life of the family. He would knock down and disorder his brothers' and sister's toys, and we had been forced to divide the nursery to keep him away from David and Andrew. He would do his best to prevent Eileen from taking an interest in Andrew and David. It was difficult for Eileen to listen to David and Andrew reading, to read to them, or to help them with their school homework. When Eileen went out shopping with the children, Bernard might throw some tantrum and lie down on the pavement. As he grew older and heavier, his tactics became harder to deal with. We were also concerned for a time because Andrew was very slow to begin talking. Was this because of the example of Bernard? We shall never know. Perhaps not, for I was a late talker myself, and we later found that Andrew had a minor speech defect arising from the structure of his mouth. Nevertheless, we were worried at the time, and wondered if Bernard was responsible.

These years, while Bernard was growing up from two to seven, were probably the worst of all. Each year he developed new capabilities, and a great number of these were very troublesome. We managed to deal with them, but we were very conscious that we were only doing so because we had the extra help about the house. We both began to feel that if he became much worse, or if we lost our help about the house, then it might be difficult to keep him at home. We had also come to feel that Bernard did not think in the same way as other children, so that going into a home would not have been so traumatic an experience for him as for a normal child. (Looking back we still feel that this view was correct, although it would not be true of Bernard as he is today.) Therefore, when Bernard was seven, we both agreed to put his name down with the City Health Department for a place in an institution. This registration in no way committed us to sending him away, but helped to ensure that if it became necessary then a place might be available.

After this decision, life with Bernard continued just as before. We certainly had no intention of his going away in the near future. There was, however, an important corollary to this decision, on which I felt strongly. Namely, that if he were going to remain at home with his brothers and sister, then we would expect him to behave properly, just like his brothers and sister. Of course, one does not expect a 5-year-old to behave as well as a 10-year-old, or a mentally handicapped child to behave as well as a normal child of the same age. However, it was clear by then that Bernard was capable of reasonable behaviour, provided he was sufficiently encouraged. It was clearly all too easy to accept lower standards of performance and behaviour, on the grounds that he was, poor chap, just a mongol. In fact, I describe in the next chapter, how Bernard's behaviour has improved enormously because we expected it to.

Chapter 9

Training Bernard

Because a handicapped child grows up more slowly, he finds everything more difficult to learn, even the everyday tasks of feeding himself and dressing himself. One has to spend time and energy teaching an ordinary child to learn these techniques, and occasionally he can be very troublesome. Even so, the effort required to train Bernard was an order of magnitude greater.

When Bernard started on solid food, at about the age of two, he had very definite likes and dislikes. We have already said that he would only accept sandwiches containing either sausage or banana, or both. At first we cut the sandwiches into small pieces, which we passed to him one at a time. The next step was to place the cut pieces of sandwich on his plate, and let him feed himself. Bernard got the idea at once. He picked up a piece and popped it in his mouth, but then immediately picked up another piece, and put that in too. By the time he came to the third or fourth piece his mouth was almost full, so a finger went in to try and make more room. Bernard was now in a sorry state, his mouth full of sandwich and finger, unable either to chew or complain. We then had to remove first his finger, and then one or two pieces of sandwich, so that he could get on with his meal.

Bernard looked pretty uncomfortable with his mouth so full of food that he could not move his jaws. Yet, as soon as his mouth was empty again, he was always ready to repeat the performance. It was quite obvious that he had not enough intelligence to realise that if he put too much food into his mouth, he could not eat at all.

Bernard eventually overcame this habit because I gave him a smack every time I saw his mouth over-full. This training took a long time, but in the end he got the message. We have the impression that his habit of putting too much in his mouth was not peculiar to Bernard, but a characteristic associated with mongolism. He certainly has an inbuilt tendency to this habit. Even today we occasionally see his mouth rather too full, and he would not have grown out of this habit if left to himself. A normal child eventually realises how to avoid difficulties, and takes pleasure in doing tasks properly, but Bernard was quite different.

There was no pleasure in teaching Bernard to eat, but it had to be done. Like every other child, Bernard needed to be taught the techniques and social graces that make up the fabric of all our lives. However, with his limited mental capacities, he could not learn very many at once. It was therefore essential to concentrate on the most basic points. He needed to be trained in *something*, so the obvious place to start was the art of feeding himself.

When Bernard was about three, we introduced him to a spoon and pusher. As soon as normal children are capable of handling these tools, they are generally pleased to do so, but Bernard was very slow at learning how to deal with them. For a long time he found it difficult, and therefore preferred to use his fingers. He was smacked, first for not even trying to use a spoon, and then, when he could use a spoon, for making do with his fingers. He eventually learned how to use both a spoon and pusher very effectively, so that on our voyage to the USA his table manners on the ship were almost above reproach.

It is a characteristic of mongols that they have rather clumsy little hands, and an extra long tongue. Therefore another habit of Bernard's at meal times, was to bend over his plate and lick up the food straight into his mouth. This habit immediately occasioned a hard smack. We have never seen this behaviour in normal children, but it lasted with Bernard for a very long time. Another variant of this easy way of eating came later when he could use a knife and fork. His head would sink lower and lower over the plate until, using his fork as a scoop, he would push his food straight across the plate into his mouth. Even today we often have to remind him to sit up straight, so that his mouth does not come too near the plate.

Bernard has always struck me as rather a lazy little boy. He is of course very backward, but quite apart from that he shows many symptoms of preferring the easy option. (Maybe this is really a sign of intelligence?) At times his mother has been satisfied with his progress, but I found myself thinking that Bernard was capable of a better performance, and we would set about teaching him a further ability. It is worth recording Eileen's view of this.

John decided when it was time for Bernard to learn to do something new for himself, perhaps learning not to stuff a whole piece of bread into his mouth, or to handle a fork, or to cut with a knife. John made sure that his knife and fork were not too big and unmanageable, and showed him how to use them. Bernard was encouraged with praise when he really tried, but was discouraged from stuffing his mouth full of bread and butter by a sharp smack.

When a pattern had been established, I would attempt to continue when John was not at home for the meal. At the beginning of a new phase of training I was often conspicuously unsuccessful. If I said 'No, you must not stuff food into your mouth', the only result was that Bernard would scream, and push and bang any plate I had left within his reach. In fact, we had more screams and tantrums at meal times than at almost any other period.

Bernard's meal-time training has continued over the years, and he has made steady progress. He started using a spoon and fork when he was three, and a knife and fork when he was nine. By the time he was eleven he could cut with a knife, but was still reluctant to practise the art. At the age of thirteen his performance with a knife and fork excited no particular comment, though of course we must remember that he still looked rather like a 7-year-old. He is still apt to give up rather easily. If the meat is hard to cut, he tends to try to tear it. If the butter is hard, he soon gives up trying to spread it. If he is very thirsty, he will drink a whole glass of water in one great gulp, and then sit looking very uncomfortable. However these episodes are now only occasional lapses from an otherwise creditable performance.

More important than his improved manual dexterity, is the fact that he now has a clear idea of what is expected of him. He knows what is the accepted way to behave, and makes some effort to act in this way. Recently he was having difficulty in cutting some fried bread, because he was not using his knife properly, and was attempting to divide the bread by a pulling and tearing action. I looked at him and said: 'Give him another fork, instead of a knife, so that he can tear it properly.' At this, Bernard began to cut the bread normally. There was no need for anyone to explain to him how to do it: he knew, and just required encouragement. We also recall one lunch-time, not so long ago, when Bernard became very cross with David. Bernard's mouth had sunk lower and lower towards the plate, and it looked as if he were going to begin a direct transfer of his lunch straight from the plate into his mouth. He was asked to sit up, and did so, but then David gave a mimic performance of eating his own lunch by this method. Even though Bernard had been about to behave this way himself, he appreciated the situation sufficiently to be most annoyed by David's comment.

Bernard's efforts to dress himself make a very different story. Until he was about five he had to be dressed completely, but then he made serious attempts to dress himself. When he got stuck he was helped, but we left him to try until he had come to a halt. He was always willing to make the attempt, and there were never any screaming fits or tantrums.

At this time, Bernard was able to watch Maureen, who was growing up towards his mental age. She, too, was learning to dress herself, and this must have helped Bernard. They were bathed together as soon as Maureen could sit up in the bath. After the bath they were dried, cuddled, played with, and dressed, with the other either in the bath or standing watching. By the time Maureen was four she could dress herself completely, and Bernard, then nine, was also getting the hang of the matter. Vests, pants, round-necked shirts and jumpers had been mastered, although trousers were more difficult, and socks and shoes still unsolved problems.

Our visits to Chapel Farm each Easter provided a powerful incentive for Bernard to dress himself. He wanted to go out each morning to watch the milking which began at 6 o'clock, but Eileen was not prepared to get up so early to dress him. For many years he had to stay behind while his two brothers crept noisily out of the cottage into the farmyard. He was first allowed to join them at the age of eleven. He still needed a little help in the final stages of dressing; this was usually provided by David or Andrew, but on one or two mornings Eileen had to get out of bed because of moans and groans from the next room. There, she found a disconsolate Bernard, only partly dressed because of some difficulty which had arisen after David and Andrew had gone out thinking that he was virtually ready. By the following Easter, Bernard was able to dress himself adequately without his brothers' assistance. He would finally put on his wellington boots and outer jacket, and then go off to the milking. He returned for breakfast at about 8 o'clock, looking the picture of dishevelment, with boots on the wrong feet, jumper back to front, zip undone, vest and pants showing, and (as he had just left the cowshed) covered with a fair sprinkling of cow dirt. However, by the following year he could dress himself tolerably well.

As with most children, he has found socks and shoes the most difficult part of dressing. Even today he is still not very good at getting socks on properly, and the heel is often seen at the front of the foot. He still cannot deal properly with shoe laces, but can fasten and unfasten the buckles of his sandals. He is less good at remembering to put the sandals on the correct foot, and does not worry too much on this score. If one reminds him, he realises they are wrong, and can change them over. He finds shoe laces difficult because of his small and rather clumsy fingers. For this reason it was not until he was thirteen that he learned to do up the toggles on his duffle coat. He can now do this well, and is also just about able to deal with big buttons on an overcoat or mackintosh, although small buttons still give him trouble.

It is worth pausing for a moment to ask why Bernard behaved so differently in learning to dress himself and in learning to eat. The answer is probably not hard to find. Unless you dress yourself in the accepted manner you feel uncomfortable. If your arms and your head do not go through the correct holes in your vest, shirt and jumper, then you are very much aware that something is wrong. Bernard, slow-witted as he is, knows when he is not comfortable. There are also right and wrong ways of putting on pants and trousers. On the other hand, it is not so obvious that socks should go on in a particular way, and you are not terribly uncomfortable if the heel is not quite in the right place.

Feeding yourself is quite a different matter. The food is there before you on a plate, and you have two hands and ten fingers which seem designed to take the food straight from the plate into your mouth. They do the job quickly and it is all very easy. If you have podgy little hands with clumsy fingers you find holding a fork, a spoon, and a pusher very difficult. They twist round in your hand, and unless you hold them just the right way, the food may slip off before it reaches your mouth. It all takes time, it is very frustrating, and life would be so much easier if we used our hands. Of course, if Daddy is there, one has to make a bit of an

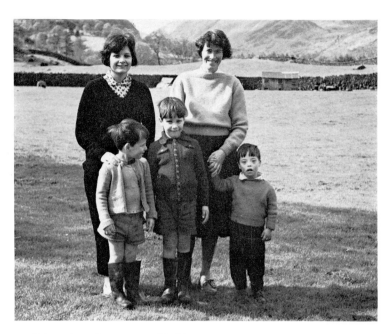

9 Bernard at $5\frac{1}{2}$, a group with Tess

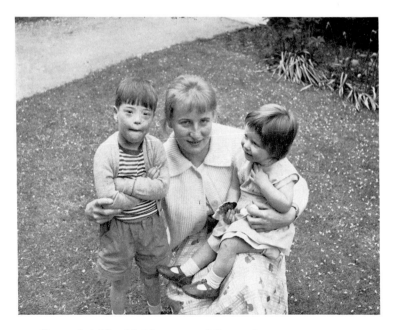

10 Bernard at $6\frac{3}{4}$, with Maureen and Irmgard

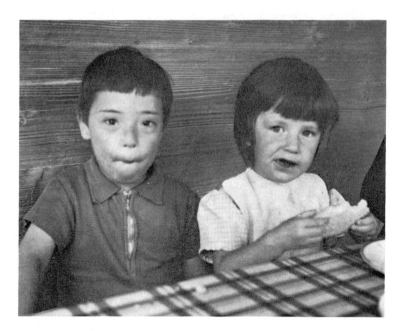

11　Bernard at $7\frac{3}{4}$, with Maureen

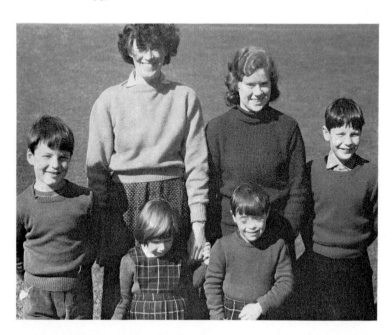

12　Bernard at $8\frac{1}{2}$, a group with Annelyse

effort otherwise there is a smack; but if Daddy is not, then Mummy's smacks are not so hard. Mummy is easier going than Daddy. Back to the easy life. Anyway, what's all the fuss about? What's wrong with using fingers?

It would have been quite impossible to explain to Bernard what is meant by social acceptability, to explain that if he wished to go out with us, then he must behave as other people behave. (Of course, Bernard would have had much less trouble at an earlier stage of civilisation when knives and forks and spoons were unknown!) It seems fairly clear that the tantrums at meal times arose because we were asking Bernard to do something which was fundamentally difficult for him, and for which he did not see any real need or reason. Even today he needs the occasional reminder to sit up and eat his food properly, although he always makes a good job of dressing himself.

While on the subject of dressing, we should say something about the choice of clothes for Bernard. A normal child generally looks attractive in most clothes. One notices not so much his clothes but that his eyes are bright, alert and full of mischief; he may also be dirty and untidy and quite careless in his dress. Life is so exciting for a small boy, there is so much to do, so much to learn, such fun to have, that he has no time for the mundane tasks of washing his hands, keeping tidy, and worrying about his clothes. With Bernard matters were rather different: his little face was rather dull, and the type of clothes which had looked attractive on David, and later served equally well for Andrew and Maureen, looked positively hideous on Bernard.

Another reason for not passing down David's and Andrew's clothes to Bernard was that he was a continual fiddler with buttons. If Eileen gave him an ordinary shirt with buttons down the front, he fiddled until every one was undone. He would then pull at the buttons until they came off, and would finally twist his fingers in the button holes making them larger and larger. T-necked shirts that fastened on the shoulder with one or two buttons received similar treatment. He would fidget and twist and pull until the neckline was completely ruined, the seams torn, buttons off, and holes enlarged. The same thing happened with button-up pyjamas, except that at night he had a longer period without supervision, so by the morning his pyjama tops were sometimes in a bad way.

When buying clothes for Bernard, Eileen had also to take account of his shape. Bernard was not a well proportioned little boy. He has always had a fat tummy, and hardly any waist, so it is not easy for his trousers to stay up. He really needs to wear braces, but they involve buttons or other gadgets that just ask to be fiddled with. In fact, an entirely different type of wardrobe had to be bought for Bernard. Shopping took longer, because Eileen had to search for round-necked T-shirts, and pyjamas and jumpers which fastened with no buttons. In addition, the colours and style had to be more carefully selected than for the other children. Eileen made some of her best finds in the girls' departments of the stores!

Another point which had to be borne in mind when buying clothes was Bernard's habit of fiddling with himself if given the least opportunity. If he was in short trousers, and sitting down, his hand would go up into his trousers. He did it rather absent-mindedly, and stopped when told, but as soon as he became bored, up went his hand again. The easiest way to deal with this was to buy him long trousers, and he has lived in them most of the time.

A more marked characteristic when he was about fourteen, was to play with himself in his sleep, and he had a tendency to take his pyjamas off in bed. Even in the depths of winter we might discover him at 11 o'clock with nothing on. We woke him up, made him dress himself, and gave him a ticking off. He then behaved for a couple of months, and we all repeated the procedure.

Another habit was to push both his hands into the back of his trousers, thus revealing a display of Bernard's bottom, sometimes an embarrassing addition to the public scene. This was a favourite trick which often needed attention. If at home, Eileen would pull his trousers right down, smack his bottom, and push them up again; if out of doors we would give him a scolding. Eventually he slowly improved, and grew out of the habit. It was an absent-minded habit, and Bernard was always surprised when we drew his attention to the matter.

We now turn to toilet training. Some handicapped children give their parents a very hard time for several years before they agree to be trained. We were fortunate with Bernard in this respect, although we had our troubles, particularly for a year when Bernard was about 4 years old.

At first we made no attempt to introduce Bernard to toilet training. He picked up new ideas so slowly, that we did not expect him to be fully trained before four or five, even at best. We therefore kept him in nappies all the time. After three years he remained dry during the day, but was wet at night. More important, he generally became dirty during the night. As Andrew was also untrained for most of this time, one of Eileen's main impressions of the period is of an endless washing of nappies.

The position changed for the worse when Bernard's intelligence began to develop at the age of about four. He discovered how to take off his dirty nappy when it woke him up during the early hours of the morning. He immediately discovered that he had something to play with on the grand scale. Many books on the training of mentally handicapped children emphasise the stimulation that these children can receive from painting and the graphic arts. Bernard is no great painter, but we suspect that few activities have given him so much satisfaction as using his dirty nappies to decorate the floor, the walls, the windows, his cot, his Dinky toys, and anything else he could lay his hands on. It was quite a sight for Eileen when she saw his first efforts in the graphic arts. It was also a lot of work for her. Bernard had to be taken up to the bathroom, undressed and washed from head to foot, then dried and kept warm. Meanwhile Eileen returned to the nursery with disinfectant, rubber gloves and buckets of soapy water, to deal with the floor, walls, windows, cot, and everything else.

These episodes did not occur every morning, but about once a week. They were very tiresome, and we were not at all successful in discouraging them. We tried smacking him, without any effect at all, for he forgot all about the matter in a day or two. We tried taking him out of nappies and giving him a potty, for he knew how to use one in the day time. Here we scored what is sometimes called a 'limited success'. He got up and used the potty in the early morning, but then turned it upside down, and played as before. We now had a pretty good idea of when all this occurred. It was generally about 4 o'clock, but neither of us felt inclined to get up at that time, and make some attempt at supervision.

The state of affairs when we went to the USA with Bernard coming up to the age of five, was just as described above, but in our first two months in the USA he was trained quite quickly by the efforts of our niece Anne. She was young and determined, and had sufficient energy to wake up between 4 and 5 o'clock each morning, and march a protesting Bernard to the toilet, where she sat him on the lavatory seat until he performed. As like as not he would do nothing, but get down, and make towards bed. Anne then gave his bottom a hard slap, and sat him back on the seat.

He did not like this at all, and protested loudly, but well before two months were out, he was accepting the new régime. Moreover, the hour when he first woke up moved forward from 4 o'clock to 6 or 7, and by the time that Maureen was born in September, Bernard was completely trained. Afterwards there was the occasional lapse, but he never gave us any real trouble on this score again. Eileen is probably right in thinking that this training went through with much less commotion than if Mummy had been in charge!

We have spent some time in describing the difficulties Bernard had in feeding himself, and in toilet training, because these matters are almost certain to bulk large in the upbringing of any mentally handicapped child. However, as we have stressed these difficulties, it is only fair to Bernard to point out that his behaviour has now reached a very satisfactory standard. We can take him anywhere with us, on any occasion, and know that his behaviour will be reasonable. We should also mention that his training in some matters went very easily. He learned to wash and bath himself, while being bathed with Maureen. Maureen made her first attempts, and Bernard copied her. Hence, as Maureen was able to wash herself from the age of three onwards, Bernard could do the same from eight onwards. Of course, Bernard is not always ready to use his ability to deal with dirty hands and face, but then neither were his brothers and sister.

Finally I mention a few other examples of Bernard's training going very easily. Both Eileen and I like to concentrate on what we are doing when driving the car in traffic, and the children have learnt to keep quiet on these occasions. Keeping quiet is not Bernard's strong point, especially in a busy street, with lots of interesting things to see. Nevertheless, Bernard has always been well behaved in the car, even when alone with Eileen, for he enjoys his car rides. If he shows signs of misbehaving, Eileen has only to say 'Be quiet, or you will not come out with me again.'

(When Bernard was small, our car had only two doors, so the children on the back seat were in no danger of falling out. When we acquired a car with four doors, we changed the door handles at the back, so that they could only be opened from the outside. Thus with the children sitting in the rear there was no possibility of their opening the door by accident.)

We have a number of books in the house and all the children have been taught to respect them. They were not allowed to handle our books until they showed that they could treat their own properly. When they were toddlers they were not allowed on their own into the lounge, where most of our books are kept. These rules were always accepted by Bernard, and he never damaged any of our books. He may come into the lounge occasionally and fiddle with the record player, but he does not touch the books.

Bernard has also respected his brothers' and sister's books. He has his own collection at the bottom of a bookcase in his bedroom, and he keeps them in good condition. He likes to look at them early in the morning when he wakes up, and likes someone to read to him each evening. He is perfectly safe with books of all sorts. Lest this account appears too good to be true, we must admit that until about three years ago he was a bit of a trial to his brothers and sister over their school exercise books. Bernard did not realise that empty pages must stay empty, and sometimes if a pencil was lying around he made his own peculiar writing marks, and the page would be covered with Bs. He saw his brothers and sister writing in their exercise books each evening, and probably wanted to do likewise. On the other hand, when he brought his own exercise book home from school, he was most indignant when Eileen suggested that he should mark the nice clean pages by trying to write something in it.

As one more example of easy training, we mention his one-time habit of grinding his teeth. Although both Eileen and I had heard the expression 'to grind one's teeth', neither of us had any experience of what this meant. However, when Bernard was about 8 years old, he made the matter very clear to us. He began to grind his teeth in his sleep, and occasionally made a noise as if he were putting all his strength into forcing one set of teeth over the other. At the time he was sleeping in a cot in our bedroom, and this noise was loud enough to wake us up in the middle of the night. We would shout: 'Bernard, you're grinding your teeth.' We made sure that he was awake, and had heard us, and then went back to sleep. Sometimes a second shout was necessary, sometimes not, and the habit died away in a year or two.

Chapter 10

Bernard in Public

In this chapter I describe some of our experiences, or more often Eileen's experiences, in taking Bernard about in public. His earliest visits were to the shops, where he always seemed at his naughtiest. An ordinary child dislikes standing around in a shop; he cannot see over the counter, and much of what interests his mother is incomprehensible to him. Hence it was hardly surprising that Bernard often 'played up' on these occasions.

Matters did not improve even when Bernard discovered something which really interested him in the shops. At the age of about six, he discovered the till where the money is kept. No two shops have the same sort of till, some ring a bell, others have counters which fly up, all have knobs to push, and a drawer which flies open. The till had a great fascination for Bernard, who has a definite mechanical bent. Given the least opportunity, he would whip round to the back of the counter, and play with it.

Bernard's various activities in the shops would not have been so bad had it been possible to tell him to stop. However, for a period of about ten years, he objected strongly to any verbal reprimand. In reply, he would sit down on the spot, and scream. Eileen was always aware of this possibility, and was forced to plan her shopping expeditions so as to avoid this kind of trouble.

Life would have been much simpler for Eileen if she had left Bernard at home when she went shopping. However, she felt that this would be tantamount to saying that Bernard would always have to be considered separately, and treated differently. If we wanted Bernard to be a full member of our family, we had to give him every opportunity to grow up and develop, as far as he was able. We had to see whether or not he could be trained.

Difficult as Eileen's task was, it was not a hopeless one. She had something very definite to work on. She knew that Bernard's behaviour with me was really very good. I only took him shopping occasionally, but when I did there was never any sign of trouble or tantrums. Eileen also knew from the way Bernard behaved at home when I was present that he was perfectly capable of behaving himself if he wished. She was well aware that Bernard's behaviour with her was often not very different from that of an ordinary little boy being thoroughly naughty. All that was necessary was that Bernard should behave as well with Eileen as he did with me!

From an early age, visits to the local shops often involved a skirmish between Eileen and the shopkeeper on one side and Bernard on the other. At this time, Eileen received much sympathetic understanding and co-operation from the shopkeepers on her regular round. We are most grateful to these kind people who have watched Bernard's progress with interest, and are now pleased to see how much he has improved. They have played an essential part in Bernard's training.

When Eileen was having trouble in a shop, she used to emphasise that Bernard was being naughty with her, and that he could at times behave perfectly well. Quite frequently a kind shopkeeper would make some face-saving remark, such as 'Bernard's not exceptional, a lot of children like to come to the back of the counter. Most children like to play with the till.' 'Oh, do they?' Eileen would reply gratefully, although fully aware that none of her other children had done so, neither could she recall seeing other children up to these tricks. All the same, these little face-saving remarks were much appreciated.

Everybody on the regular shopping round soon realised that Bernard had to be treated kindly but firmly. If he was greeted too kindly, or in too friendly a manner, he would soon be at the till or up to some other mischief. In fact he interpreted an over friendly manner as permission to play as he chose. Eileen still recalls a day, when Bernard was nine, and she was out with him in another part of Oxford. She needed some particular item, and went into a shop hitherto unknown to her. The girl assistant greeted her, and was particularly friendly to Bernard, 'How are you, my love?' she said with a smile. Bernard needed no second invitation, and ran round to her side of the counter. Eileen's heart sank, for she knew that there would be trouble when they came to leave. She was right, but first there was trouble over the till. Bernard pushed all the wrong keys, he shut it, he opened it, and generally misbehaved. Eileen had to go round and pull him out from behind the counter, and there was quite a struggle. Eileen left, dragging a screaming Bernard, and regretting that she had ever come into the shop!

However, by the time he was fourteen, the results of Eileen's efforts were clearly visible. She could then go shopping with Bernard without fear of there being a scene. Bernard was even able to do a little shopping by himself, thanks to the prolonged efforts of Eileen and the local shopkeepers. We must admit that he still sometimes had his off days, but he did not sit down and scream when asked not to do something. He might stop walking, and refuse to budge, and say 'No', but Eileen dealt with this one by walking away and leaving him. He had sufficient intelligence and innate caution not to go on to the road, and eventually followed behind, sulking. After a few minutes he came up to be cuddled, and to say 'sorry'. We must admit too that he loved riding on lifts or escalators, and he always found it a terrible wrench to leave such exciting places!

In many ways training Bernard while out shopping was no different from dealing with an ordinary child. He had to be taught not to touch things, not to walk round to the back of the shop, and so on. Although Bernard has a low IQ, he has considerable curiosity as to how things are put together, and is a great fiddler. As an ordinary child, he would have been troublesome in a shop for a time, but being handicapped he took much longer to learn how to behave. However, as Eileen has remarked, 'You have to go through a particularly trying and embarrassing period for about five or six years. You have to put up with this, if you want to train the child to behave in a socially acceptable manner. For the alternative is that you do not take him out at all.'

When Bernard was about seven, Eileen started to take him to church with the other children. Just as Bernard had to be trained to go shopping, so he had to be trained to go to church. Eileen felt strongly that, as one of the family, he should join her and the other children at church. I was very sceptical. I thought that he would probably be a nuisance to everyone in the church, and make his own unwanted contributions to the service. It seemed very doubtful that he could understand what was going on, or obtain any benefit from the service. However, events were to prove me wrong.

There is a small Carmelite chapel quite close to our house, so as a preliminary to going to services, Eileen began to call in with Bernard on the way to the shops, to get him used to the building and to teach him to genuflect. Bernard would go into the chapel readily enough, but sometimes had to be dragged out, as from the shops. However, after a few visits he was ready to go to mass on Sundays. The preparations of Eileen and the children leaving the house were not always peaceful. Quite often Andrew was screaming because he did not want to go, while Bernard who did want to go, was screaming in case he was not allowed to. Eventually Bernard stopped screaming and Andrew dragged himself along the three minute walk, as far behind as possible.

Once in the chapel, Andrew would start to fidget, and push against whoever was next to him. Eileen would therefore sit between Andrew and Bernard to keep them apart. Then Maureen was beyond Bernard, and wanted to sit beside Mummy, so she and Andrew changed places. This did not always produce peace, for if Andrew was not next to Mummy there might still be trouble. However, the only really disastrous incident occurred when, during the shuffling and fidgeting, Maureen fell over, hit her head, and began to scream.

Eileen had chosen to start Maureen and Bernard off at the Carmelite chapel, because it was a small church where it was easy to beat a hasty retreat should the occasion demand. (In fact this was only necessary the time Maureen fell over.) The chapel also had the advantage of anonymity, as the Carmelite nuns sat out of sight, and could not see the antics of our family. The congregation numbered no more than fifteen or twenty, most of whom were very sympathetic and kind. Even so, Eileen felt tired every Sunday morning.

Looking back over those early days at church, Eileen suspects that she may have been over anxious about the behaviour of the children. They were probably no worse than the average family. Bernard was never worse than Andrew, and Eileen thinks none of the children was as bad as she had been as a child. One of her earliest recollections is of a High Mass, when she made her way up and down the length of the church, underneath all the pews. A mother is probably far more conscious of distractions provided by her children than anybody else. For example, Eileen was concerned that the priest at the chapel might have been disconcerted by the various shufflings. However, when she got to know him better, she found that he was slightly deaf, so that it was doubtful if he was ever aware of the children!

After a year or two, for reasons quite unconnected with Bernard, Eileen started to take the family to the morning mass at Black-friars, the Dominican friary in the centre of Oxford. At that time Maureen was about four, Andrew about seven and Bernard about eight, so Eileen had three children all inclined to be more or less difficult in church. Blackfriars is the theological house of studies of the Dominican order in England, and not a parish church. The con-gregation at the 9 o'clock mass was quite small, but on the other hand the choir stalls were filled with the students wearing their long white habits and black cloaks. The mass itself was very colour-ful, a High Mass said by three priests in brightly coloured vest-ments, and an organ with the organist in view. Because there was so much to watch, Eileen suddenly found that all three children were quiet and interested.

Bernard would stand, sit, or kneel, in a very well-behaved manner, although his movements seldom synchronised with every-one else in the church. Eileen soon learned that he reacted very negatively to suggestions that he should conform, so he was left to sit when everyone else was standing, and to stand when everyone else was sitting, even though this meant that he stood throughout the sermon. In fact, Eileen generally managed to give her attention to the sermon without being much distracted by the children, although she often breathed a sigh of relief when it was safely over. A few people in the congregation were probably well aware of Eileen's misgivings; at least they smiled at her encouragingly on her way in and out of church.

When Bernard was nine, he started going to church without his mother. His school began to arrange visits for the children to two nearby churches, according to the wishes and denominations of the parents. Bernard, with others of his school-fellows, went once a week to the Shoppers' Mass in the nearby Catholic church. These visits obviously went off well, for in the following year Father Neil Smith started to teach Bernard and one or two other boys to serve mass. Reports of Bernard's progress came back from the school, and after another year, when Bernard was eleven, Eileen was invited to attend the service and watch him in action. She saw him kneeling beside his teacher, who told him and his friend John when to go to the altar. Once there they both knew what to do, but Bernard's performance was not up to standard; he was rather silly and giggly, probably overcome by seeing Eileen in unfamiliar surroundings.

Shortly afterwards, various rearrangements took place at the school, and there was no longer time to make the visits to church. It seemed a pity to Eileen that Bernard's serving activities should be brought to an end, and she had the good fortune to arouse the interest of one of the Dominican priests, Father Charles Boxer. For about eight weeks, Charles said mass at Blackfriars each Saturday morning, so that Bernard could go on learning how to serve. Bernard wore his ordinary clothes, the mass was said in one of the side chapels, and the congregation consisted of Eileen and Maureen, and two friends.

Right from the start, it was obvious that Bernard had been well trained by Father Smith. He knew what to do with hardly any prompting. He rang the bell at the right time, he brought the wine and water correctly, and he knelt or stood devoutly at the foot of the altar. Admittedly, there were occasional lapses. While standing, he might suddenly bend over and put his head between his legs, or while kneeling he might decide to see what went on under the carpet. However, he gradually improved and made steady progress. Indeed, after about six Saturdays, he became over-confident. Then, in typical Bernard fashion, he was rather naughty, and started to tell Charles what to do. It seemed that for the moment Bernard had learned all it was profitable to teach him!

Two or three months later, the morning High Mass at Blackfriars was replaced by a simpler mass, designed for parents with young families. Father Geoffrey Preston, who was in charge of the arrangements for this service, suggested that Bernard should now serve mass in front of the full congregation. Bernard was quiet and attentive during the whole service, and knew exactly what to do. For his first mass, Eileen dressed him in his vestments but subsequently he allowed Geoffrey to do this for him. He has now served at masses with other priests, at masses with three priests, and at masses where the procedure has been different from usual.

Sometimes, of course, things do not go quite smoothly. Eileen recalls one morning when there were three priests officiating at mass, not all of them known to Bernard. His last duty was to fold a linen hand-towel, lay it over two small glass bottles that stood in a glass bowl, and carry the bowl from the altar to a side table. It so happened that the linen towel was not as stiff as usual, so that when folded it drooped down towards the water in the bottom of the bowl. Bernard refolded the towel, replaced it on the two glass bottles, and picked up the bowl, but the towel still drooped down. Once more, Bernard refolded the towel, and again it drooped down. It was now pretty obvious to Bernard, and everyone else, that it would always droop. Bernard looked round wildly towards Eileen, who mouthed at him that it did not matter, so with a sigh of relief he carried away the bowl and the drooping cloth.

Besides Bernard's regular weekly appearances at the shops and at church, we also recall a miscellany of assorted outings. Eileen would take him to watch his brothers and sister play games at their school. Bernard thoroughly enjoyed going, but soon tired and refused to stand still for very long. He would also object strenuously if Eileen talked to one of the masters or to another mother, but the answer to this was simply to stand in a part of the field where there were not too many other people. Occasionally Eileen took the children to play hide-and-seek on the little wooded hill at Shotover near Oxford. They all ran around and Bernard enjoyed himself as much as anyone, without attracting any undue attention.

Bernard made his first visit to the theatre at the age of nine, when Eileen took him with the other children to see *Cinderella* at Christmas. Previously we had not considered him reliable enough to sit through a $2\frac{1}{2}$ hour show without becoming restive and wanting to go home. His behaviour showed that we had been too pessimistic. He was enthralled by the pantomime, and his behaviour was perfect. At the interval, he ate his ice cream, and went off to the toilet with David, all without incident. Subsequent visits to the pantomime have been equally successful, and he particularly enjoys slapstick comedy. He does not go very frequently to the cinema, but has twice seen *The Sound of Music*. Each time he sat motionless from beginning to end.

When Bernard was almost twelve he was taken on a new form of treat, a train ride to Didcot alone with our Dutch girl Emmie. The journey had been carefully chosen. It was not very far, so Bernard would not become bored. The train turned round at Didcot and came straight back to Oxford, so there was no tedious wait between trains. Emmie reported that the outing was uneventful, and that Bernard had been as good as gold; he had obviously enjoyed it very much. Later the same year Eileen took Maureen and Bernard up to London for the day. They went by train, and travelled on the underground and the escalators. They had lunch in a fish-and-chip shop, and then looked round the Zoo, where the high-light was the chimpanzees' tea-party. Both Bernard and Maureen enjoyed everything they did, and were no trouble at all. Bernard's promoted to the dodgems (under careful supervision!) By the time to the St Giles Fair held in Oxford each September. He loved the roundabouts, but until he was about 8 he had to be lifted bodily off when his turn was over. Then from nine onwards he was promoted to the dodgems (under careful supervision!) By the time he was twelve, he was advanced enough to visit the Fair alone with David, who was happy to look after him.

When Bernard was eleven Eileen managed to take him on a successful visit with Maureen to the local museum. Maureen wanted to go, and it was necessary to take Bernard as well. They did not stay very long, but walked fairly quickly through the whole building, so that Maureen could see what she liked best. It was apparent that Bernard was not particularly interested in any-thing, and Eileen held him firmly by the hand. No doubt he felt rather put upon, but even so they were all able to look at a fine model of a large Roman villa for quite a time, and he seemed to enjoy this as much as Maureen. In company with his brothers and sister, he has also visited a number of cathedrals and other old buildings which we like looking at on our holidays. Provided our visits have not been unduly lengthy, and we take care to avoid this, Bernard finds his new surroundings sufficiently interesting that he is prepared to keep going for as long as the other children.

Occasionally Bernard was invited out to tea at the home of one of his school friends. Unlike David, Andrew and Maureen, he had no friends who lived near enough for him to visit without our making detailed arrangements. We fear, however, that he was not the ideal guest. He enjoyed his tea, but then instead of playing with his host, he preferred to sit down and watch the television, no doubt feeling that he must make up for not having a set at home. Often, he was only willing to play chasing games, of the kind where everyone gets wilder and wilder, and more and more out of control. The two friends he visited most, Andrew and Debby, played with their toys, and would have been happy for him to join in. Bernard, on the other hand, would only watch them, or agitate for the television to be switched on.

The position was much the same when his friends came to tea with us. They were generally happy to play with his toys and with him, but Bernard tended to ignore them. When Maureen was smaller, she played with the guests, but Bernard stayed with Eileen as she prepared tea, and showed no desire to entertain his friends at all. Bernard did not shine on these occasions, compared with his friends Andrew and Debby. In fact, we sometimes thought that Bernard only wanted his friends to come to tea, so that they would invite him back, and give him a chance to watch the telly.

The picture we have just drawn of Bernard presents him as a rather unsociable chap, but this is not the whole story. He has been on good terms with our next-door neighbours, and we have already mentioned how attached he is to the sons of the house at Chapel Farm. We are told that at school he got on well with everybody, and had no particular enemies. This, we gather, is more than could be said for every child at the school. We were also told that Bernard appeared sensitive to children worse off than himself, and took a sympathetic interest in anyone who appeared unwell.

Finally we mention Bernard's birthday parties. Eileen first started on this venture when Bernard was 6 years old. She was a little doubtful about having a party of his school friends, as she was not sure how the other children would behave. Bernard at this time could be extremely difficult, and she had visions of all the children being nonco-operative all the time. Fortunately, she knew his teacher very well, so Eileen asked if she would come to the party, and also help select those of Bernard's friends who would not be too much trouble.

Six children came to the party, and it was very fortunate that the teacher was there as well. Not because they were naughty or troublesome, that was no worry at all, but because they were extremely shy and quite lost in this break in routine. However, they all ate their tea, and seemed to enjoy it. The following year the party was repeated, but without the teacher, although Eileen checked the invitation list with her. The party was again uneventful, and the children were not so shy.

This pattern went on for several years. After each party Eileen used to think how easy it had been. David was always very helpful, and our current *au pair* girl came and generally brought a friend. The children were often easier to deal with than some who turned up to parties for David, Andrew and Maureen. Certainly none of the parties was as disastrous as one that Eileen gave for David a long time ago, and still remembers. Then Eileen became over confident. She thought she knew most of the children in Bernard's class, and which were his friends. So when he was twelve, she did not check the list of guests with his teacher, and she had a frantic party. Two of the boys became nearly uncontrollable, one spent the whole time trying to escape from the garden, the other went screaming round the garden in a very wild manner. The party had to be terminated, and all the children bundled into the car, and taken home. The two naughty ones were then very abashed and sat quietly in their seats, obviously well aware that the party was all over because of them. The following year the well-tried procedures of previous years were again applied and all went smoothly as before.

Chapter 11

Behavioural Problems

Writers on mentally handicapped children sometimes remark that they may be 'over-active', and exhibit 'behavioural difficulties', but very often give no clear indication of what is involved. We assume that these terms include the temper tantrums which for so long were a constant part of life with Bernard. As the most troublesome and difficult part of training Bernard has been in dealing with these tantrums, we spend most of this chapter on this one point.

The task of dealing with tantrums fell almost entirely on Eileen, because Bernard virtually never put on these scenes either for me or for our *au pair* girls. The treatment varied according to where Bernard was at the time, who was about the house, and whether Eileen was tired or not. If Eileen was somewhat tired, she might not handle him as skilfully as usual, and the tantrum would really develop. If she was more alert and energetic, then it might be a small tantrum. As Dr Down wrote eighty years ago, 'discretion will often be the better part of valour.' Although Eileen could often control the size of the tantrums, there seemed to be no rhyme or reason in when they would commence. It was, however, pretty certain that something would go wrong each afternoon.

About once a week, there was a scene when he came off the school bus. Sometimes he refused to come off at all. At other times, he would come off quite happily, shut the coach door, and then hang on to the door handle. Eileen would grab his hand, and un-twine it quickly as the coach started to move away. He next sat down on the pavement, cross-legged, and refused to move, Eileen then had to drag him across the pavement into the house as quickly as possible. Once in the house, he was either left in the

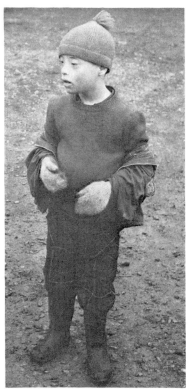
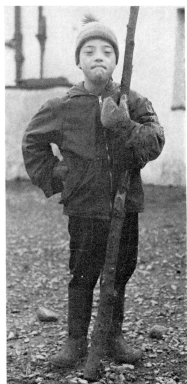

13 At Chapel Farm, Bernard 10½

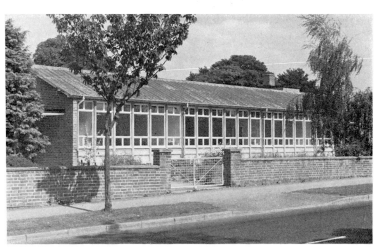

14 Bernard's school

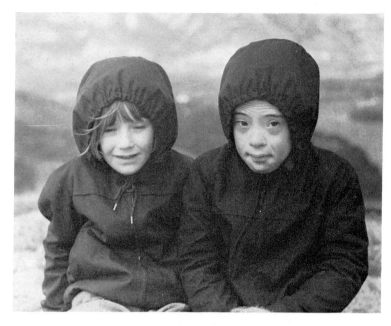

15   On Catbells, Bernard is 10½ and Maureen 5½

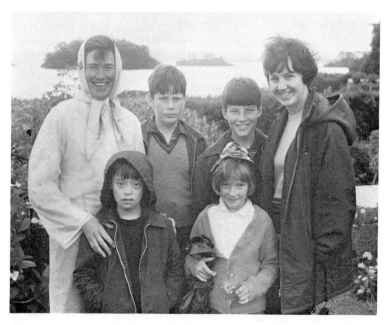

16   Bernard at 11¾, a group with Mira

hall to simmer down, or passed over to the *au pair* girl, who diverted his attention to something else.

When it was time for Eileen to prepare tea, Bernard would watch, and all was generally quiet and peaceful. Bernard might even assist with the preparations, and help lay the table. Then Eileen would ask David, Andrew and Maureen to come for tea and wash their hands. As Eileen made the final preparations for tea, they grudgingly washed their hands. At this stage Bernard usually said 'No', and disappeared under the kitchen table. The only way of getting him to the tea table, was to pick him up, and sit him in his chair. He did not go very willingly.

Once at the table, he behaved himself, more or less. His table manners on these occasions would be well below his best perfor- mance, but if Eileen recalled the merits of discretion over valour, the meal might pass fairly quietly. One of Bernard's favourite tricks at this time was to sulk throughout the meal, and only start eating when everybody else was getting down from the table. Often when I came home after tea, I found him having his meal all by himself.

When tea was over, Bernard could be relied upon to throw another tantrum, if he thought that Eileen was spending too much time playing with the other children, or indeed if she spent any time with them. Eileen would then pass Bernard over to our foreign girl, who would play with him in another room. If not removed, he would have made it quite impossible for Eileen to give her attention to the others.

Eventually it was time for Bernard to have his bath and go to bed. He would usually refuse to go to the bathroom, and have to be dragged up the stairs. He would not co-operate in undressing, and was frequently dumped screaming and kicking into the bath. He would then subside and enjoy his bath, but might refuse to come out. Eileen would try to get him out peacefully by threatening to throw cold water over him, and by sometimes actually throwing the water. On other occasions, he had to be pulled out screaming and struggling. The screaming and struggling continued as he was dried and dressed. If Eileen let go, he would promptly sit down on the floor and refuse to budge. Finally, still screaming and struggling, he would be half dragged, half carried, into our bedroom and put into his cot. As Eileen knelt down to say prayers with him on such evenings she was quite exhausted.

What were the underlying causes of the tantrums? Bernard undoubtedly wanted to get Eileen's attention, and he certainly succeeded when he was totally unco-operative and screaming. Other mothers have told us that their handicapped children were also reasonable as long as all the attention was being given to them, but as soon as Mother dealt with their brothers and sisters they set up a considerable commotion. When Bernard was only a baby, Eileen had been warned by her parish priest that a handicapped child could be very demanding on the mother's time, and that this would be detrimental to the other children. It was only now, however, that Eileen fully appreciated what 'demanding' could mean!

Although there was very often a fuss when Bernard thought he was being neglected, there were often occasions when he objected violently to being given too much attention. He has always been rather set in his ways, and indeed sometimes reminds us of a fussy old gentleman. Changes in routine, or even a break in one activity, are unwelcome. A request to come and have tea quite often sets off a tantrum. These tantrums were, of course, all the more likely if the request was to do something unwelcome. If some of his clothes were on back to front, or if we could see his pyjamas showing below his day clothes, any suggestion that he should put matters right generally met with a very poor reception.

There was often a certain amount of trouble when it was necessary to wash Bernard's face, and clean his nose and ears. He did not like having his face washed, and the job was often a lengthy one. Sometimes two people were needed, one to hold his hands out of the way, the other to wash his face. His standard remark on these occasions was to complain, we think without much justification: 'Hur me, hur me', that is: 'Hurt me, hurt me'. In a like manner, the business of combing and brushing his hair had to be kept as brief as possible.

One of the principal difficulties of dealing with Bernard on these occasions was the impossibility of explaining to him why various things were necessary. For example, you turn off the water taps when the basin is full, because otherwise the water will flood over on the floor. You wash your hands and face before a meal, especially if you have been playing outside in the sandpit, so that you do not become ill. For a very long time, these complicated ideas and explanations meant nothing to Bernard. As far as he was concerned, there were just too many 'Dos' and 'Don'ts', for apparently no reason. All too frequently, he made his views on these occasions abundantly clear to us. Eileen had only to say 'Bernard, you have too much food in your mouth', and trouble had arrived.

People often suggested to us that one of the causes of the tantrums was Bernard's frustration at not being able to make us understand what he was trying to say. We feel that there might be something in this, but not a great deal. The tantrums were at their worst before he attempted to say anything other than 'No'. Yet, even then, we were perfectly certain that he understood what we said to him. When he was in a good mood, or if I was about, he responded to requests and questions in a way that showed he understood and could reply. As soon as he tried to talk, and made very weird noises, we could generally understand what he was trying to say; Maureen in particular was an expert interpreter. There were certainly some occasions when he became frustrated because we could not understand him, but on these occasions he did *not* throw a tantrum.

As we have already said, the most difficult part of training Bernard was to cope with the almost daily tantrums. Occasionally, on the more trying days, Eileen lost her temper with him and gave him a smack, such as his brothers might have received on similar occasions. He was then upset by the smack, and also genuinely upset at making Mummy cross. She too was upset, feeling guilty at having lost her temper. However, it was noticeable that Bernard's behaviour then improved markedly, at least for a short while.

Eileen had a much worse time over tantrums than either I or our *au pair* girl. Bernard hardly ever made a scene when I was present, or when he was alone with the girl. The reasons for this must be quite complex. One factor was certainly that I was much stricter with him than Eileen. When we had been training him to eat properly at table, I had been present at most breakfast and lunchtimes. As soon as he started doing something he knew he was not allowed to, he received a sharp smack on his hand. He disliked this, and mended his ways. He was also well aware that if I asked him to do anything, I seldom let him get away without doing it, or at least making some attempt to do so. I saw very little of the tantrums with which he plagued Eileen. Very occasionally I would come across Eileen and Bernard either after a shopping expedition, or after one of his worst tantrums at home, and find Eileen very upset by his behaviour. His bottom was then soundly smacked, and he behaved better, for a time.

It is sometimes suggested to us that Bernard's behaviour has not been very different from a normal child's save that he has taken longer to grow up. This is not our experience when we compare him with his brothers. There were certainly times in their early days when they threw tantrums and were similarly punished, but these were rare occasions which quickly passed. They were never of such intensity, or caused Eileen so much upset. In contrast, Bernard's tantrums were an almost daily occurrence.

Sometimes when I was absent at tea-time, Bernard would be in a dreadful state of agitation, purple in the face with fury, and there would be a knock on the front door. He instantly scurried off to sit wherever he ought to be, and as I came into the room all was peace. Sometimes I did not knock at the front door, but would walk down the side of the house, past the dining room window, to the back door. Usually, everybody but Bernard saw me pass, and waited with some amusement to see Bernard's 'quick change' act as I came in. Sometimes, when I was out and Bernard was in a tantrum at tea-time, David would disappear out of the room. Shortly after there was a knock at the door, Andrew would say 'That's Daddy', and peace would automatically descend. Unfortunately, as Bernard grew older, he learnt to see through this deception.

Almost certainly, I had fewer tantrums with Bernard because I was stricter with him than Eileen, but this was not the whole story. His behaviour with all our *au pair* girls was also quite different. He behaved with them very reasonably, and almost never threw a fierce tantrum at them. In fact, through all the years, we have never had a serious complaint against him from any of our girls; they all say how fond they are of him. Of course, he always gets off to a good start with them because he is very friendly when they first come to the house. They arrive, feeling perhaps somewhat strange in a new country, and Bernard goes along to keep them company. He talks with them, and generally tries to be helpful. He is in fact pleased to see them, and is almost always on very good terms with them.

I have already mentioned that David can take Bernard about, and finds him well behaved. Once when Bernard was about fourteen, Eileen was out with him and Maureen, and he was being somewhat awkward. Instead of walking home, he wanted to sit down at each bus stop, and wait for the bus. He was being rather obstinate with Eileen, but in the end was jollied along home by the efforts of Maureen. As they reached home Maureen said 'You know, Mummy, I can handle Bernard better than you, don't you think so?' Eileen could only reply 'Yes', for Maureen had certainly been responsible for getting him along the half mile to the house.

There seems little doubt that it is in the nature of things for children to prefer to take it out of their mothers. At any rate this was the case with Bernard. We must remember, of course, that Bernard saw very much more of Eileen than of anyone else. It was therefore much more difficult, or even impossible, for Eileen to be either very strict, or very friendly, for the whole of the time. If anyone was going to receive a tantrum, she was the obvious target. Again, Bernard would often go for a walk with me very cheerfully, whereas if he had gone with his Mum he would probably have grizzled all the way. Of course this type of behaviour is not peculiar to Bernard. We can recall expeditions on holiday a few years ago, when either I, or Eileen and I, went out walking with David or Andrew. The boys would come along with me happily and cheerfully, but on very similar excursions when Eileen was present they were sometimes disheartened and discouraged. This behaviour was very reminiscent of Bernard's performance with his Mum, although on a much reduced scale.

As the years went by, Bernard's behaviour improved, but only very slowly. It was also beginning to be a race against time. The pattern of Bernard's tantrums remained pretty much the same, but by the age of nine or ten he was getting appreciably stronger. Although still very much undersized, see *Plate 13*, he was getting heavier and more muscular. Eileen was finding it more difficult to pick him off the floor at tea-time, and sit him on his chair. He would refuse to stand up, and go limp if she tried to lift him. When under a table, he would hang on to a leg with both hands and refuse to budge. When eventually Eileen dragged him out, he would try to kick and punch her, all the time screaming 'No'. I almost never saw this performance, but I recall one afternoon when I happened to see him through the window coming off the coach towards the front door. He usually looks as if butter would not melt in his mouth, but on this occasion he looked very bad-tempered and fierce, and gave the impression of having it in for somebody. Unaware that I was at home, he marched into the hall, and advanced on Eileen both arms flying round as if to punch and pummel her. At this stage he saw me, said 'Oh!', and all was peace!

It was now getting on for ten years since Bernard was born, and Eileen was much less emotionally inhibited by the fact that he was handicapped. It was becoming quite clear that poor weak little Bernard was in danger of becoming unmanageable. To have accepted unsatisfactory behaviour now would have ensured that he would become unmanageable when not much bigger and stronger. This was not just a vague fear, for many handicapped children are brought up at home to about this age, but then become so difficult that they have to transfer to an institution.

If Bernard was to remain at home, he would have to behave reasonably. He would have to learn not to punch and kick Eileen when she made a reasonable request. It was also quite clear to Eileen that Bernard now had a perfectly good understanding of what sort of behaviour was expected of him, and that if he chose he could behave well. For instance, if Bernard had been naughty when out with Eileen, I would sometimes have a word with him before he went out with her the next time. I would tell him that I would ask Eileen whether he had been a good boy while out, and that if he was naughty he would be in trouble. This reading of the riot act invariably ensured that Bernard behaved himself.

Now that the position was becoming clear to Eileen the next time Bernard made one of his more outrageous scenes at tea-time, she did not lose her temper. She took him off to the nursery, put him over her knee, and spanked him really hard. After he had been cuddled and comforted, he returned to the tea table and to a much better pattern of behaviour, at least for a few days. There followed a period of six months, when Bernard was spanked by Eileen about once a month; by the end of this time his behaviour had begun to improve, and it has continued improving ever since.

The severity of Bernard's tantrums decreased, slowly at first, but steadily. By the time he was eleven, Eileen was finding him more amenable, easier to handle, and less likely to stage a sit down strike. There were fewer disappearing tricks under the table, and fewer absolute rages. He continued to say 'no' forcefully, and there were reversions, but life became easier, and there was not such a difference in his behaviour when I was and was not about the house.

By the time he was fourteen, his behaviour was by no means perfect, but was usually quite reasonable. To give one example, Eileen noticed that he had put too much butter on a piece of bread, and asked him to take some off. In the past this would have created a first-rate tantrum, and even on this occasion he took exception to Eileen's comment. He made his protest by looking sulky and pushing his plate away from him across the table.

Nobody took much notice of this. He sat there looking sulky for a minute or two, and then pulled back his plate, and started eating again. Another welcome sign was that he quite clearly did not like seeing his Mummy cross with him. Indeed one of his more clearly enunciated phrases at that time was 'Mummy not cross?'

It has always seemed to us that Bernard is often just plain naughty, like other children. A good example of this occurred at about the age of fourteen. Bernard was on very good terms with our next-door neighbours, and on occasion was to be found talking to them in their garden. However, one day, Mrs Green mentioned to us that he had developed the habit of going uninvited into their house, switching on the television set, and sitting himself down in front of it. We agreed that this was not the way for Bernard to behave, and we said we could discourage him. 'But', said Mrs Green, 'perhaps you can't stop him. He may not understand that this is wrong.' Sometimes Bernard is so slow to grasp an idea that one can well understand Mrs Green's remark, but we drew his attention to the matter. The following afternoon Eileen returned home to find Bernard with a dustpan and brush, filling the pan with clippings from the privet hedge which were lying about the front garden. Then, when the dustpan was full, he emptied the contents over the wall, to land right in front of Mrs Green's front door. No doubt he was saying to himself, 'That will teach her to tell tales on me!'

Although we have talked mostly about temper tantrums, there is one other behavioural problem that has given us serious concern. Bernard has a very mechanical and inquisitive bent of mind. As I have said before, he likes fiddling with mechanical gadgets, and finding out how they come to pieces. He is only too willing to fiddle with anything, to find out how it works. This intellectual curiosity is very commendable, but one has to make certain that he does not take an electric light switch to pieces and put his fingers in, or leave the gas stove turned on. When he was younger, it was well-nigh impossible to explain to him that these devices were very dangerous.

Our methods of dealing with this security problem have varied over the years. Many of his first exploratory expeditions were made by getting up early in the morning, at about 5 o'clock, and exploring the house on his own. When he was about five we moved his cot from the nursery to our bedroom. He then did not wake up so early, or if he did, he soon went back to sleep again. Later, when he slept in the same room as David and Andrew, we resorted to locking the doors leading to the kitchen and the bathroom where he could do most damage.

Although the technique of keeping Bernard under our eyes, and of locking doors, worked quite well, it was by no means a satisfactory solution. If Bernard was going to grow up in the home, then he just had to learn to recognise which things were really dangerous. He would not learn this by any policy of isolation. Therefore as soon as his understanding seemed sufficient, he was allowed to wander round the house, in the hope that he would not do anything too stupid.

When he was caught doing something really dangerous, like fiddling with an electric plug, or playing with a gas tap, he was first given a smack and a ticking-off. The ticking-off was generally received with a very jaundiced air. His face and mouth were pulled into a characteristic expression, which we took to mean 'Oh dear. I don't see why they're making such a fuss.' We were left wondering if he had learnt his lesson. In fact, a relatively mild ticking-off seemed to produce little effect. It was often only a matter of one or two days before he was fiddling with something else equally dangerous. At this stage, I put him over my knee, and spanked him hard. He would then confine his fiddling to less dangerous objects, at least for a few months. His behaviour has slowly improved over the years, but as we describe later it still gives us occasional cause for concern.

Chapter 12

Doctor and Dentist

We have often been told that mongols are less healthy and robust than normal children, but Bernard gives little sign of being much different in this respect from his two brothers and sister. Almost the only difference was that until he was about seven he became very low spirited and miserable when he caught the occasional cold. However, the colds always seemed to clear up after a normal period of time. Apart from these he was hardly ever ill. One summer his face became swollen, and this was diagnosed as mumps; he was kept in his cot for one day, and was soon running around again.

Although Bernard has enjoyed remarkably good health, he has had a fair number of visits to the doctor, for a variety of quite normal minor matters, such as septic spots, and cuts and bruises. More often than not, these visits have left us feeling thankful that they do not occur very frequently. Bernard is nearly always quite prepared to talk to the doctor, and to fiddle with all his interesting and strange pieces of equipment, but he is not prepared to do much else.

There is usually some trouble at his yearly medical examination at school. He objects strongly to having a wooden spatula placed on his tongue. His first reaction is to grab the spatula and throw it away, and second not to open his mouth. He will allow his chest to be examined with a stethoscope for a short while, but will then try to grab at it during the remainder of the examination. At his last school medical, Eileen did not go as she thought he might behave better without her, alone with his teachers in his usual surroundings. In fact, he was as unwilling to co-operate as usual.

On one occasion, Eileen took Bernard to Dr Stewart for an ear inspection, as we wondered if he was hearing as well as he should. All went well until Dr Stewart took out his device with a light bulb at one end to inspect the ear. Bernard did not want the bulb anywhere near his ear, and it was only with difficulty that he was persuaded to keep still long enough for it to be seen that both his ears were blocked with wax. The treatment was obviously to syringe his ears, but Bernard viewed the syringe and the small tray to collect the water with extreme suspicion. He knocked the tray out of Eileen's hands with a loud 'Naw', and withdrew as far as possible from the doctor. The whole operation was obviously not possible, so instead Dr Stewart prescribed ear drops for Eileen to administer at home. This she did each night, with no trouble at all, and eventually all the wax came out. She then had to return to Dr Stewart for him to check that the ears were clear. This time, however, once Bernard had assured himself that there was to be no syringe, he did not mind the light being put inside his ears.

Given Bernard's reaction to the suggestion that his ears should be syringed, it is not surprising that we both well remember the day when he had to be taken to the casualty department at the local hospital. When Bernard was about 8 years old, he caught his finger in the hinge of a door, so that the very tip of the finger was nearly severed off. We took him down to the hospital, where his screams immediately resulted in his jumping right to the front of the queue. He was very frightened, and it took Eileen and three nurses to hold his hand and arm still while the doctor stitched his finger up, without an anaesthetic. By the time he returned home, he was utterly exhausted, and soon went off to sleep. After recounting an episode such as this, friends sometimes remark: 'Well, an ordinary child would have been very upset.' True, but Bernard was even more upset.

Not surprisingly, visits to the dentist also produced difficulties. He was quite willing to talk to the dentist, and to ride up and down in the dentist's chair, so that his first visits passed off quite well. Trouble only started the day the dentist found a tooth that needed filling. The dentist actually succeeded in doing some drilling, and inserted two wads of cotton wool into Bernard's mouth while he was preparing the filling. Bernard found these uncomfortable, so he promptly took them out, and threw them on the floor. Eileen held his hands, as another was inserted. He spat this out, and tried to get out of the chair. However, the dentist eventually persuaded him to stay put, and to open his mouth long enough for the filling to be inserted after some fashion.

At the next visit, four months later, Bernard eyed the drill with great suspicion. As soon as the dentist took it in his hand, Bernard was wriggling out of the chair. This was one of the few occasions when his behaviour was no better at all when I was present! After one or two similar visits we usually tried giving him a sedative half an hour or so before the appointment. This helped, provided that the dentist was running to schedule. One morning, in particular, Eileen watched the effects of the sedation gradually wearing off, so that by the time they went into the surgery, Bernard was alive and kicking as if he had had no sedation at all.

Until very recently, it was quite hopeless to try to explain to Bernard the reason why his teeth needed treatment. He saw no point in the whole business. As a result, none of his teeth was ever filled properly, so the time arrived when he began to have tooth-ache and the only treatment was to extract a tooth. This was done under gas one Saturday morning, and Bernard was terrified at the sight of the anaesthetist, his assistant, and their equipment. He started to scream as soon as they brought out their face masks, continued to scream until he lost consciousness, and then continued to scream for another fifteen minutes as soon as he came round. Before the next extraction, a year later, when he was about eleven, Eileen asked if he could be given a sedative beforehand, but was told that he must have nothing at all to eat or drink for the previous twelve hours. This second extraction was if anything worse than the first, and Bernard did not stop screaming for the next thirty minutes afterwards. To complete this little scene, the anaesthetist then asked Eileen why she had not given him a sedative.

A year later Eileen was told that four milk teeth needed to be extracted, so she asked if this could be arranged in hospital under a general anaesthetic. Our dentist was co-operative, and in due course Bernard and Eileen were visiting a well-known dental surgeon in his surgery at the local hospital. By this time Bernard had an active dislike of our own dentist. The mere sight of his house was enough to discourage him, and he was now very reluctant to open his mouth for the dentist to even look inside. However, in the hospital surgery he was first allowed to wander round the room, and the watchful nurse in attendance was told to let him play. When he was quiet, the surgeon sat him on the chair, and gently looked at his mouth. Bernard was like a lamb, opened his mouth wide, and kept it open. When the inspection was over, and they said goodbye, Bernard returned to the surgeon and kissed him goodbye!

A month later, Bernard was admitted to the Churchill Hospital on a Sunday afternoon, and the teeth were extracted on the Monday morning. Eileen spent all Monday afternoon with him but he was still very much under the influence of the anaesthetic. She collected him on Tuesday morning, when he was fit, and well and happy. She asked him what had happened. He put his hand over his mouth and said: 'No'. 'Oh,' said Eileen, 'no gas?' 'No.' Then he made a great demonstration of injecting his arm with a big jab. 'Did that hurt?' asked Eileen. 'No,' he replied. Fortunately his second teeth have not given much trouble so far, but we do not look forward to the time when further treatment becomes necessary.

Finally we mention two points about Bernard which have often struck us. The first is his long reaction time to pain. If he bangs his head, or hurts his finger, there is a very long pause before he cries out. At least it seems a long time, and is certainly of the order of two or three seconds, whereas an ordinary child would shout immediately. The other point, which we mentioned in chapter 6, is that his whole personality seems to run in cycles, as if at times he is powered by quite different fuels. For a period of perhaps a few weeks he will look duller and less intelligent than usual, and will actually be so. We say to ourselves that it is one of Bernard's dim periods. Then he perks up and seems to be brighter and more intelligent than ever before. We suspect that his metabolism is influenced by some biochemical processes, which at present are not at all understood.

Chapter 13

At School

Bernard began going to school when he was about 4½ years old. At that time, his accomplishments were comparable with those of David and Andrew when they had started at a nursery school soon after their second birthday. We had no great hopes that Bernard could receive any formal education, but thought that attending a playgroup would be a useful experience. In addition, his sessions at school considerably reduced the task of looking after him at home. Bernard was put on the school bus at 9.15 a.m., and he came home at 3.45 p.m., each Monday to Friday.

It is only since 1971 that Bernard's school has been officially called a *school*, the Mabel Prichard School. Until 1960 it was known as an occupation centre, and then for several years as a training centre. These changes reflect the growing realisation that the possibilities of training and teaching mentally handicapped children are much greater than was thought in the past. Eileen and I have always referred to the centre as a school, even when it was officially an occupation or training centre, and we referred to the lady in charge as the headmistress. Bernard was in fact going to school, like his brothers and sister, albeit a school of a different kind.

Until 1971 the Mabel Prichard School was run by the City Health Department, but then the responsibility for all such schools was transferred to the Department of Education and Science. The school has been steadily developed and improved over the years, and appreciably so during the time that Bernard was attending. It now has accommodation for about sixty children of all ages up to about sixteen. They are looked after by the headmistress and, at the moment, six other teachers.

The school is housed in a pleasant modern building on the out-skirts of the city *(Plate 14)*. Running along the front of the building, are four large classrooms, while behind and at the sides are a set of ancillary rooms, including a large kitchen, dining- and staff-rooms. There is also another classroom with a set of ancillary rooms, know as the Special Care Unit which we mention below. The building is surrounded by large lawns, with swings, a climbing frame, a paddling pool, and a kitchen garden in the background.

Most of the fifty or so children are divided between four classes. Their classrooms are not very different in appearance from the rooms one might find in a normal school. However, if one saw them unoccupied, one would assume that the children were not much older than six or seven. In addition to the four main classes, there is accommodation in the Special Care Unit for children under 5 years of age, and for children with physical handicaps in addition to mental handicap. On the average there is one teacher to each class of about ten children.

The aims of the school could hardly be put better than in one of the yearly reports of the City Medical Officer of Health.

> The training of the pupils at the school is organised so as to help their social adjustment as much as possible. For the youngest children there are play activities to help develop their manipulative skill, and training in personal hygiene and simple social matters such as how to behave at table. Every effort is made to enlarge the children's vocabulary and as they grow older they are taught to count and to do simple sums. They learn to recognise letters and some simple and important words and to copy letters and to write their own names. They learn to recognise coins and learn their different values.

Of course these aims must be approached slowly. We have described above how Eileen and I had to spend time training Ber-nard in the many simple skills that most children pick up very quickly. The average child of five knows how to look after him-self, communicate with others, play with other children, and has some manual and physical dexterity. These skills are the essential foundations on which all other progress must be built. However, if a child has a severe mental handicap, it is quite certain that he will not have learnt these skills by the age of five. Therefore, the training at the school must first deal with very simple tasks.

When the children arrive off the coach, they have to remove their coats, and hang them up on their own peg. This in itself is the first lesson of the day. In the middle of the morning, they have a drink of milk, which must be set out, drunk, and then cleared away. They must wash their hands before lunch, and clean their teeth afterwards. Then, after a rest and a play, it is time to get down to the difficult business of putting coats on and making ready for the coach to take them home. The routine at the school is in fact reminiscent of that at a nursery school for ordinary children of a much younger age.

One of the main tasks of the nursery school for ordinary children is to encourage them to open their eyes, to look around, and to use their imagination. Likewise a vital part of the training of all mentally retarded children is the encouragement of interest, and of the urge to learn, which is much feebler than in normal children. They need stimulation at first on a very modest level, for example simple and colourful toys, simple musical sounds, or just the talk between teacher and child. Physical exercises, such as walking, running, climbing stairs, jumping, ball games, riding a tricycle, all play their part. Some of the children at the Mabel Prichard School have swimming lessons, and have gained proficiency certificates. If children can do these things reasonably well, their opportunities for contact with other children are greatly increased. These contacts will then stimulate the child's power of communication and the acquisition of other social skills.

As the child becomes older more sophisticated methods are used. One of these methods came to light when Eileen was visiting the school one evening for a parent-teacher meeting. One corner of a classroom was called a 'blue corner', and contained lots of blue articles, a book, some Dinky toys, a doll's bed, a doll's dress, all looking neat and attractive. In addition, there was a book, the Story of Ping, which looked familiar. 'What's that doing there?' thought Eileen. Apparently Miss Wallis, Bernard's teacher, had asked her class to bring something blue to school with them, and Bernard must have collected the book just before going off to school, without saying a word to anyone. The blue corner was an exercise in teaching the children to remember to do something, and then to perform the simple task itself. It was a variant of an earlier exercise when Bernard took a bag of stale crusts each day to feed the birds from a bird-table made by himself and Miss Wallis.

The children are taught to count by means of practical activities. Each day one child, from the top class, is sent round all the class-rooms with a board, to count the number of children in each class. He then collects the correct number of milk bottles and delivers them to different classrooms. At other times the children are sent on little errands around the school to find, say, ten bean bags or ten small bottles. We imagine that Bernard saw some point in these activities, and made a good job of them. At home, he enjoys laying the table for a meal for seven people and manages with no trouble. On the other hand we cannot see Bernard showing any enthusiasm for writing down numbers, counting coloured discs, or any other activity that involves sitting down in front of a book. Nevertheless some of the children in his class were quite good scholars, and they were encouraged to do as much as they could.

We have the impression that some parents think that the school does not make enough effort to teach the children the rudiments of the basic skills of reading, writing and arithmetic. This is a difficult point. These skills are tremendously important, even at a very modest level. It is obviously very useful to be able to read, and to recognise simple words such as 'push' and 'pull', 'danger' and 'stop', 'Ladies' and 'Gentlemen'. It is equally useful to have enough arith-metic to set out the right number of plates for dinner, or to make simple purchases. On the other hand, the children often show little enthusiasm for any sort of formal work. Some can be taught to read, and understand simple introductory reading books, but others have great difficulty. Some, like Bernard, find it difficult, and are also very reluctant to make the necessary effort.

Although Bernard liked Eileen to read to him from his books, he had no wish to read himself. She said to him one evening, 'Wouldn't you like me to teach you to read for yourself?' His answer was quite clearly, 'No jolly fear'. Yet even Bernard can be persuaded to take an interest in reading and writing. For some months Bernard carried a thick hard-backed notebook, his diary, to and from school. At the end of the afternoon, Miss Wallis wrote a short account of Bernard's day at school. He brought it home, and showed it to Mummy so that she would know what he had been doing. Before he went to bed, he made sure that Eileen wrote down an account of his activities at home. He was always

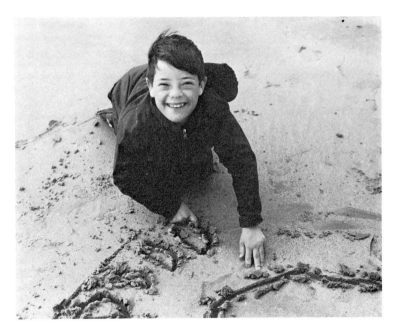

17 Bernard on holiday, aged 11¾

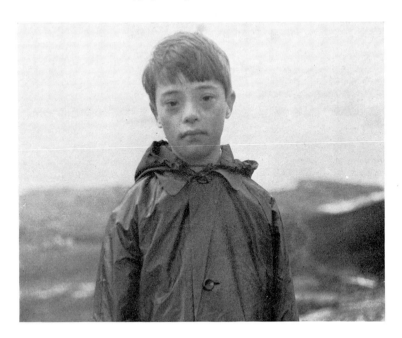

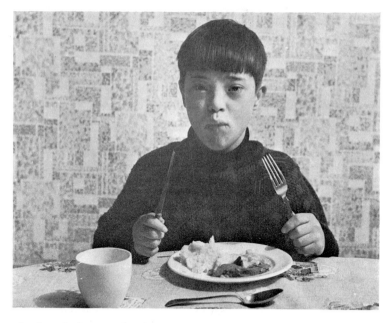

18 Lunch-time, aged $12\frac{1}{2}$

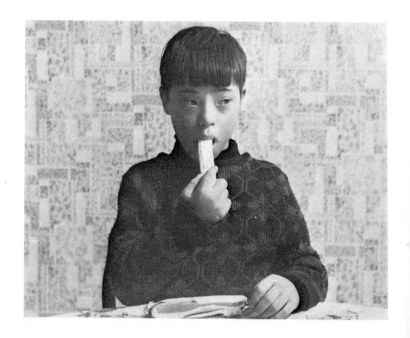

most insistent that Eileen and Miss Wallis wrote their accounts, and that Miss Wallis read Mummy's latest entry as her first task each morning.

The diary had more effect than might appear at first sight. Bernard often wanted to take up some particular activity, so that Miss Wallis could record it in the diary. Hitherto, he had not shown much interest in learning to write. He could draw a rather shaky capital B, but not much more. He realised that he too might write in the diary. At any rate, his writing, such as it was, began to improve. Bernard is often quite willing to work away on all sorts of things, provided he does not realise that his activity can be called work.

In the end we may have to admit that many of the children will have very limited ability in reading and writing. We must therefore remember that a great number of useful and essential every-day jobs either call for no knowledge of the 3 Rs, or can be so arranged. Bernard played a useful part at school by helping to sweep the floor, by helping other children to put their coats on, and by fetching and carrying things generally. On one occasion, the children moved on from making hand-print paintings to making foot-print paintings. At the end of what must have been a very messy session, all the children were left with dirty feet, and Bernard was put in charge of the washing operations. He was most insistent that everybody washed their feet, even those who were not at all keen on the idea. We only learnt about this, when we noticed a pair of extremely dirty feet as he went to bed that evening. He had forgotten to attend to his own! (After several frustrating minutes, Bernard was able to make Eileen understand that he had been painting with his feet. We only heard that he had been supervising the washing of the other feet the next time we saw his teacher.)

Besides learning from their teachers, the children also help each other. For example, Bernard was particularly friendly with two boys, John and Joe, of about his own age, both of whom could talk much more than he. Bernard could understand nearly everything that was said to him, and could go on an errand and do what he had been asked to do. His two friends on the other hand were not so reliable, they might get lost in going from one classroom to the next. So if Bernard and Joe or John went together, Bernard saw that Joe went to the right place. Then Joe, with Bernard's prompting, delivered the message, collected what was required, and the two walked back to their classroom. We suspect that

Bernard chose his friends so that they could speak for him.

As another example of how the children interact with each other, we recall that Bernard has always made a habit of asking 'Why?' rather too frequently, while his friend, Debby, used to say 'Why?' to absolutely everything. One day, Bernard realised that this was rather pointless, and took a hand in the proceedings himself. When Debby said 'Why?', Bernard went up to her and said 'Why?, Why?, Why?, Why?, Why?, Why?'. At first Debby answered as if the 'Why?' were a real question, but then everything she said was greeted by the same word 'Why?'. After a relatively short course of this treatment Debby stopped saying 'Why?'. As far as we can make out, she and Bernard are still good friends!

Our picture of the school, so far, has been that of a happy nursery school, but with the difference that the children are much older than usual. There is another aspect, however, which we should mention in fairness to the teachers. Handicapped children can at times be very awkward. As long ago as 1887 Dr Down wrote of mongols:

> Another feature is their great obstinacy—they can only be guided by consummate tact. No amount of coercion will induce them to do that which they have made up their minds not to do. Sometimes they initiate a struggle for mastery, and the day previous will determine what they will or will not do on the next day.

These are strong words, but they certainly applied to Bernard at home during the tantrum period we have already described. We feel pretty sure that, from time to time, all the teachers at the school have to cope with some difficult problems.

Bernard was very awkward at the age of thirteen when his favourite teacher Mrs Corrigan left to attend a year's training course, and was replaced by Miss Wallis. One day he threw the work which the other children were doing all over the floor. Another day, after nothing in particular, he spat at Miss Wallis and tried to kick her, something he had given up doing at home for several years. Miss Wallis took him to the headmistress, Miss Forshaw, in disgrace. This was enough for Bernard, who then apologised to Miss Wallis, and was his good little self by lunch-time. Another time he threw some cards on the floor, after he had been asked to put them away. So Miss Wallis said 'Pick them up'. 'No.' 'Pick them up before I count three otherwise you will not go out into the playground at play time.' Bernard waited until Miss Wallis counted three, and then picked the cards up. But he was not allowed out into the playground, and he knew that Miss Wallis would be firm on this point. Despite his liking for the playground, he preferred to assert his independence.

The aim of the school is to train the children so that they can take part, to a greater or less extent, in everyday life. In order to get them used to the outside world, the older children are taken on a series of visits which have included the railway station, the cattle market, the fire station, and the police station. For some years the most important of these activities was the yearly holiday, when about thirty of the older children were taken off for ten days at the seaside. They lived in a private hotel run by an understanding proprietor, looked after by four or so of the teachers, whose own visit could scarcely be called a holiday! At the same time some day excursions by coach were usually arranged for the children unable to go to the seaside.

Bernard went to the school seaside holiday for four years. He enjoyed them very much, but his first visit turned out to be more of an exercise in social training than we expected. Before his first holiday at the age of $10\frac{1}{2}$, he had been looking forward to going away to the seaside; he had his bucket and spade and swimming costume all ready for days beforehand. He went off to school with his grip of belongings very happily. One week later, when Eileen collected him at school, she found a changed little boy. He was very subdued, and hugged Eileen as soon as he saw her. As they drove along the main road in the car, he suddenly put both arms round Eileen's shoulders to hug her again. At home, he was very quiet, and did not become his usual noisy self for another month. Looking at him, you would have thought he must have had a horrible time. Yet one of the parents who had been on the holiday told us that he had been very good and had enjoyed himself. We were reminded most strongly of Bernard's reaction when he first went away from home for a weekend while we were in the USA, as described in chapter 7.

Nevertheless, when holiday time arrived the following year, Bernard was eager to go again, but he was able to tell us what had been worrying him. A good week before he was due to go he started to pack, but he also said 'Ba- ba- ba?' 'Of course you're coming back,' said Eileen, as she took all his clothes out of the suitcase and returned them to the drawer. The next night he began packing again, but this time he was stopped before the case was full. He was obviously looking forward to going, but would he come back? That was the great question. When the day finally arrived, Eileen brought his grip downstairs to find him twisting his handkerchief round and round into an ever tighter thread asking, 'Ba- ba- ba-?' 'Yes, yes, yes, you're coming back. We've only packed a few of your things, most of your clothes are still here.' In the end he went off quite happily, peace descended on the house, and a week later a happy little boy returned home. The following year he was more concerned about whether his best friend would be going with him.

Other important links between the school and the outside world are made through the interest of various groups and organisations. Often as a result of hearing a talk on the work of the school, people have thought how they could best help its activities. A small church group in a nearby village visited the school, and then organised various fund-raising activities on its behalf. The headmistress sometimes addressed the pupils at the local comprehensive school at morning assembly. These pupils have visited the school, have given a party for the children at Christmas, and have been invited back to tea in return. Bernard's school has also invited two groups of old-age pensioners to tea in return for kindness received from others at Christmas. The children made all the cakes and sandwiches, and entertained and served their guests. The school is in touch with several other groups and organisations, which have included members of a nearby American Air Force base, and the Royal Navy when they were on holiday at Weymouth. Besides giving help and support to the school, these contacts also help the public to understand the problems of mental handicap.

An essential feature of the work of any school is an assessment of a child's progress. At a normal school, the principal techniques are the assessment of written work either weekly or in end-of-term examinations. The results are then summed up, more or less numerically, in a terminal report. The methods may not be perfect, but they do give some idea of a child's progress. However, they are clearly not appropriate to children with a severe mental handicap.

The assessment of a handicapped child's performance at school is very important. This is not so much because it tells the parent what the child has achieved in the past, but because it indicates to the teacher what areas of training call for particular attention in the future. However, it is only recently that much attention has been given to the problem of how best to assess a child's progress. The well-known IQ, or intelligence quotient, tests have been used for a long time to give an indication of a child's innate ability. A score of less than about 70 is an indication that a child may be more suitably educated in an ESN (Educationally Subnormal) school. A score of less than about 55 is an indication that he would be better cared for at an SSN (Severely Subnormal) school like Bernard's. The IQ test, when administered by a trained psychologist, is certainly a very useful guide and classification. Of course, it goes without saying that such a classification must always be subject to reassessment. For example it is a simple matter to arrange for the transfer of a pupil from Bernard's school to the ESN school, if it appears that the pupil would profit from more advanced work.

The IQ test is, as we have said, a test of a child's innate ability. By and large, we do not expect it to change greatly as he grows older. It is therefore of little use as an assessment of the progress of a child's training. This is best done by keeping records of what tasks and abilities a child has been able to perform at each stage of his career. One method of making such an assessment is to use the Gunzburg progress chart (see Bibliography) which lists 120 simple operations, arranged in groups and subgroups. All the operations are of a definite and down-to-earth nature, for example, washes face more or less adequately (not necessarily behind ears), can count mechanically ten objects, goes on simple errands outside the house, can cut with scissors, plays co-operative team games and obeys rules. By the time one has put a cross or tick by 120 such operations, one has set down a fair picture of the child's achievements.

The results of one particular assessment are displayed on the chart itself, which consists of a set of concentric circles, which are each divided into a dozen or so segments. Each of these segments corresponds to one operation, the simpler operations being located on the inner-most circles. The chart is arranged so that segments relating to operations of the same general kind fall in the same sector of the diagram; there is one sector relating to dressing, another to number work, and another to dexterity. The results of an assessment are displayed by shading in the segments corresponding to the operations which the child has mastered. Then, if an assessment is made every six months, we expect to see the shaded area gradually spreading out as a circle from the centre of the diagram.

Three assessment charts are available, for children up to six, for children from 6 to 16 years, and for older persons. They are all similar in principle, the abilities being graded to the ages in question. The charts are accompanied by what is known as a progress evaluation index, which displays the results of periodic assessments, and also shows the average position reached by a group of nearly 400 children of the same age. The index therefore shows how a child is progressing from year to year, and also indicates if his performance is markedly less than the mean performance of similar children of the same age. It thus gives a useful indication to the teacher of where more training may be needed.

We have just mentioned that the progress evaluation index sets out the mean performance of a group of about 400 children. This does not mean that the aim of the school is to turn out all children with performance equal to the mean. There are great differences in the innate ability of handicapped children. Children may be quite accomplished in some activities, and backwards in others. The children at the Mabel Prichard School were divided into four classes, the division being made by considering several different criteria, of which age was but one. Social behaviour and ability must be taken into account if the children are to form reasonably homogeneous groups. Different children reach the same general level in different ways. Bernard was very weak on reading and writing, but was well up to the general level for his age in other ways.

No account of the school is complete without some mention of the Parent Teacher Association. The meetings of the PTA have an important part to play in the life of any school, but particularly so in schools for the mentally retarded. For many years, before Bernard could talk at all, these meetings were the only occasions when we learned what he did at school. He went away in the morning, and came back in the afternoon, but was quite unable to tell us how he had spent his time. The association also plays an important part in raising funds to help pay for excursions and for equipment for the school.

Finally the PTA also performs another task of equal importance. It provides a regular opportunity for the parents to meet each other, and discuss their children. The mothers of ordinary children spend much time discussing their children with friends and acquaintances. They do so partly because they like talking about their children, and partly in order to gain knowledge of how to bring them up. However, the mother of a handicapped child does not gain very much by talking to mothers of normal children. All too often she feels that she should apologise for the handicap of her child, and in any case is unlikely to gain much helpful advice. She can, however, obtain support and encouragement from parents who are themselves dealing with the same problems.

Chapter 14

Learning to Talk

From an early age, Bernard was well versed in the art of saying 'No', or rather 'Naw', but for a long time this was almost the whole of his repertoire. Until he was about 8 years old, 'Naw' and 'Mamma' were the only words that a stranger might have recognised. Yet all this time we had the impression that Bernard was developing his comprehension of the spoken word. Quite obviously, we would not have been able to train him at all, if he had not understood what we were saying. By the time he was eight, he could run errands for simple items, and comply with simple requests. If I was working on the car, and asked him to fetch a screwdriver, he would go to the tool box and select a screwdriver. His speech difficulties were not in understanding words, but in the more mechanical details of the technique of talking.

It was not easy to help Bernard to talk, as he had no urge to make conversation. However, meal times gave us our opportunity, for he did want his food. We did not allow him to lean across the table, and grab what he wanted. At first, he was allowed to point. Later we insisted that he added 'please', and later 'thank you'. These words came out as 'per' and 'go-goo'. Later again we insisted that he said 'bread', 'butter', and finally 'syrup'. These came out as 'ber', 'ber-ber', and 'ser'. These we accepted as it was obvious that he was trying, and was doing his best.

As a result of this encouragement, Bernard began to make more attempts to say simple words. However, he would never complete his words, so they never had proper endings. 'Wer' could mean 'where', 'when', 'why', or 'what'. 'Ber' could mean 'book', 'back', 'bus', 'bed', 'butter', or 'bread'. We could only understand what he meant by knowing the context, and then repeating possible words until we hit the right one, at which he would beam and reply 'Yer'.

A real improvement in Bernard's speech only began at the age of ten, when he started a course of speech therapy at the local hospital. The possibility of his taking this course arose through a set of fortunate coincidences. We have mentioned earlier that Bernard's younger brother Andrew was also slow in learning to talk. We eventually discovered that Andrew had a short tongue, and needed help in learning how to pronounce words. He therefore attended the speech therapy department of the hospital once a week for eighteen months, and by the time he was seven he was talking quite normally. When Eileen took Andrew up to the hospital, Bernard and Maureen often had to go with her, so Bernard happened to meet Miss Wallace who was dealing with Andrew.

Just before Andrew finished his course, the teachers at Bernard's school became concerned that some of their pupils were not talking. They felt that at least some of the children should be able to talk, and would benefit from speech therapy. The headmistress wrote to the speech therapy department at the hospital, and asked them to visit the school and have a look at the children. Therefore Miss Wallace made a tour of inspection, and Bernard was one of the children shown to her.

We first heard of Miss Wallace's visit when Eileen took Andrew for his final appointment the next day. Miss Wallace mentioned that she had seen Bernard at the school, and explained why she had been there. She thought that Bernard would probably profit from a course of speech therapy, but the speech therapy department was understaffed, and would not find it possible to visit the school. Eileen then asked if Miss Wallace could see Bernard, if she brought him to the hospital, in the same way as Andrew. Bernard was by now well known to Miss Wallace and had apparently aroused her interest, so she kindly agreed to this proposal.

During the following year, Eileen took Bernard to the hospital once or twice a week for half-hour sessions with Miss Wallace. Quite often Bernard did not wish to leave Eileen, and had to be dragged along the floor into Miss Wallace's room. However, once Eileen had disappeared, he settled down and worked well. Miss Wallace was very successful in arousing his interest, and persuading him to make the necessary effort. She made considerable use of a tape-recorder, both to keep a record of his progress and also as an inducement to good behaviour. Bernard was fascinated by the machine, and would work well, if he thought there was a chance of being taped. When the session was over, Miss Wallace would have a few words with Eileen, and Bernard would have a chat with his friend Mrs Provo, the receptionist. He usually became so engrossed in this conversation, that he could only be persuaded to leave by being dragged out along the floor!

At first, the speech therapy lessons concentrated on the recognition of a few simple words such as apple, bus, boy, girl, and then simple colour recognition. After each session Eileen was given a notebook with a list of the words that had been practised, so that she could continue the lessons at home. (She also used to send the notebook to school, so that Bernard's teacher knew what Miss Wallace was doing.) Eileen would try to get Bernard to run through his list of words, particularly at tea-time or bed-time. At this period, he was extremely reluctant to co-operate. By now he could say 'No more' very clearly, and used the phrase very often. Sometimes, he 'lost' the notebook as soon as he got home, so Eileen did not know which words to work on. The notebook was usually found after a search, but on one or two occasions it disappeared completely. Picture Lotto was recommended as both a pleasant game, and a painless way of learning how to recognise different shapes and words, but after a very short session, Bernard would be sure to say 'No more'.

Bernard's most persistent defect was, and still is, an inability to pronounce the ends of words, in particular a final s, d, t, or n. At first progress was almost imperceptible. Then, slowly, we began to understand more of the basic words in his vocabulary. Yet up to the age of twelve we were all the time concentrating on a few simple words or a few single syllables, and Miss Wallace and her successors had to use various stratagems to give variety to the large doses of practice on the same material. Fortunately, Bernard did not find the constant repetition of the same words as monotonous as a normal child would have done.

After about a year, Miss Wallace left to take another appointment. Her place was taken by Miss Doltray, who saw Bernard once a week, when they concentrated on the pronunciation of just one word. For example, she would give him practice in saying 'yes', sounding the final s. The next week it would be the turn for 'bus', and then 'up' and 'down' in the following weeks. Eileen continued to work on these words at home, but did not force him too much. It was pretty obvious that on some afternoons he came home from school genuinely tired, and could not do any more work. It was also obvious that he tried very hard at his sessions of speech therapy, for often when he got back home, he would slump down at the table for tea, and show all the signs of mental exhaustion.

Bernard did not go for speech therapy every week of the year, because at times he appeared to have reached a state of saturation, and to be making little further progress. These states, or plateaux of learning, are often observed by speech therapists and other teachers, but were very marked in Bernard. When it became obvious that Bernard had arrived at a plateau, the lessons were stopped for a few weeks, while we continued to practise the old material at home. After this break the lessons were resumed, and progress went on as before.

By the time Bernard was about 12½ years, Eileen was able to understand most of the single words he said to her. She had to do some intelligent guessing now and again, and it was usually necessary for her to know the context of the words. In his speech therapy lessons he would now say 'yes' or 'bus' distinctly, sounding the final s. At home he would also repeat these words clearly after us, but if we were in the car, and he saw a bus, he would say 'ber'. At first we replied 'bus', then later we had only to say 'Bernard', and he would say 'bus' correctly. In about a year he said 'bus' automatically, but this was still almost the only word which received the final s. However, if I happened to be looking at him, he might say a 'yes' with a great emphasis on the 's'.

About this time he began to attempt sentences, or rather to say simple groups of words. More often than not these sounded mere gibberish, and were completely incomprehensible to us all. He was aware that we did not follow him, but seldom became too exasperated when we gave up trying to understand. Sometimes it was better for us to stop trying, rather than to go on, lest he became more confused and incomprehensible.

When Bernard was about thirteen, Miss Doltray left the department, and was replaced by Miss Mills. It had so happened that Miss Doltray had not made as much use of the tape recorder as Miss Wallace had done, to Bernard's regret. It was quite typical of Bernard, therefore, that one of his first requests to Miss Mills was that she should use the tape-recorder! Bernard continued to work away on simple words, many of which became quite clear, for example, down, up, when, where, why, Andrew, Mau-Mau for Maureen, bread, bed, toilet, bus, school, church, priest, prior, more, no more, mow grass. By the time he was fourteen he was adding to his vocabulary words which we had not taught him specifically, for example 'salad oil'. He was at last beginning to construct intelligible sentences. For example, Andrew was away at a school camp, and one day Bernard asked 'When Andrew back?'

As a result of the above efforts, Bernard's power of communication steadily increased. We recall the first time he managed to tell Eileen about something which was going to happen later that day at school. We knew that the Queen would be visiting Oxford, and was passing near Maureen's school. At breakfast, Eileen asked Maureen whether she would be watching the Queen with the school, and whether she would be coming home for lunch. Maureen was not sure, but

'Quee– me Quee–', said our little Bernard.

'Are you going to see the Queen?' Eileen asked.

'Yeh, yeh', was the reply.

Bernard was very pleased with himself at having got this information over, and after breakfast he insisted on having a clean shirt. 'Quee–', he explained.

Another example of how information comes across from Bernard's monosyllables, arose recently when his teacher, Miss Wallis, asked him to bring some money to school to pay for a bus trip to the local police station. What Bernard actually said on his return home was:

'Mon.'

'Mon,' Eileen repeated.

'Mon,' repeated Bernard.

Eileen thought hard. 'Money?' she asked.

'Yeh.'

'Yes,' came automatically from Eileen.

'Yes,' from Bernard.

'Say "money",' said Eileen.

'Money,' said Bernard.

(One might think that this sort of distraction would prevent any conversation, but on they went.)

'What for?' asked Eileen.

'Coo,' he said.

'School,' said Eileen.

'Schoo,' from Bernard.

'What for?'

'Plees,' and this was clear, for Eileen knew that they were going to the police station next week.

'How are you going?'

'Bus,' and this too was clear.

'Who asked you to bring the money?'

'Mi Wali.'

Of course we are better at understanding Bernard's speech than most people. However, he can generally succeed in making himself understood to strangers, at least on simple and straightforward matters. Quite apart from speech, he has now acquired a considerable facility for putting information across by pointing and miming. When he was only eleven his activities in this line received a striking compliment from an elderly Italian gentleman during our summer holiday in North Italy. The gentleman had seen Bernard from time to time, and used to have a little chat with him, in Italian. He came up to Eileen one day, and remarked, 'You have a bright little boy, he understands Italian!'

Although it is very important that Bernard can make himself understood to strangers, there are times when we are thankful that his meaning is incomprehensible. When Eileen used to take him to his speech therapy lessons, the receptionist Mrs Provo often gave Eileen a cup of tea, to help while away the time. One day when Mrs Provo was away on leave, her place was taken by a temporary assistant, and the usual cup of tea for Eileen did not appear. Bernard was well aware of the omission, and went up to the assistant to tell her about her mistake. Fortunately, his complaints were not understood, except by Eileen! Before he could talk, we often suspected that when he was cross he would sometimes swear silently to himself. He certainly looked as if he did. Now that he can speak more clearly, we know that our suspicions had been correct! Fortunately, some of his choicer words still come out sufficiently mangled for the casual visitor not to realise their true significance!

As we said in the last chapter, it is important to stimulate the interest of a handicapped child at every stage of his training. Bernard is always very ready to take the easiest course, unless he feels the matter is of some consequence to him. Thus, he has always shown rather tepid enthusiasm for saying 'please' and 'thank you' at meals. However, he is now capable of passing on a lot of information on matters which really interest him, as was shown by an episode concerning our car.

When he was about thirteen, the clutch of the car was giving trouble, even though it had been overhauled only a little while previously. My garage excused themselves by saying that I had been 'riding' the clutch, but when I protested, this ploy was replaced by 'Your wife has been riding the clutch.' I very much doubted this, but agreed that both Eileen and I would take careful note of how we treated the clutch next time we used the car. The following day Eileen had to go out with Bernard and Maureen, and she told them that she was going to pay special attention to her left foot on the clutch pedal, and asked them to keep an eye on her. It was soon apparent that it was not her habit to ride the clutch. Well satisfied with this test, she returned home. After lunch, she happened to be sitting with Bernard beside her, and started to tell me that it was not she who had been breaking the car up.

'I was out in the car today, and checked that I did not ride the clutch,' beamed Eileen.

'Grrr, Grrr, Grrr,' said Bernard.

'Oh,' I said, 'is that the noise the car makes when Mummy is driving it?'

'Yes, yes,' said Bernard, 'Grrr, Grrr, Grrr.'

'There's no need to go on,' said Eileen firmly, for she had certainly not intended to mention these noises to me. In fact while they had been out, Eileen had slowed down to turn into a side road, and as she tried to change down from third to second gear, there was a horrid grinding noise. 'Mamma,' squawked Bernard. She moved the gear lever back to neutral and tried again, this time with more success. All went well for a little while, but then at another turn there was again a grinding noise and another squawk from Bernard: 'Mamma.' Eileen had decided that there was really no point in including this episode in her story of the car journey. Bernard, on the other hand, was very anxious to tell me about it, and had no difficulty in doing so. (In fairness to Eileen, I should say that the grinding noises came about because the garage had misadjusted the linkage between the gear lever and the gear box. Hence when the gear lever was moved in the usual way to engage second gear, the car attempted to go in reverse.)

Just as Bernard can often make his meaning clear on matters which he regards as important, he can also often pronounce a word correctly provided that he is in a state of stress. He may want something badly, or Mummy and Daddy may be making a fuss, and the result is that he gets it right. A good example of this type of stimulus occurred some time ago, while we were having tea. Bernard wanted some bread and butter, so he looked at Eileen and said 'Break-k, per.' Eileen saw that the bread was some distance away from her, but close to David. She also thought that Bernard should ask for the bread more clearly, so she replied:

'David has the bread. Look at David, and say to him "Bread please, David".'

Bernard looked sourly at Eileen, and repeated:

'Brea-k, brea-k.'

'Look at David,' said Eileen.

Bernard began to shout:

'Brea-k, brea-k.'

'If you want to behave that way,' said Eileen, 'you had better go upstairs to bed.'

Bernard turned reluctantly to David:

'Brea-k, per.'

David decided to back up Mummy, and replied:

'Brea-*d, d* not *k*.'

'Brea-*k*,' said Bernard stolidly.

'Brea-*d*,' repeated David.

By now Bernard had become tired of all this tomfoolery, and shouted out:

'Brea-dk, brea-k, brea-k. No more!'

'Let him have it, he has tried,' said Eileen.

For the next minute or two there was a pause while some steady eating went on. Then Eileen, having run out of bread herself, said mischievously:

'Could you pass me the brea-*k* please, David.'   ,

This nonsense was too much for Bernard.

'No,' he shouted, 'bad Mamma, brea-*d*, not brea-*k*.'

He had pronounced the word perfectly!

As a result of the speech therapy lessons, and of our efforts at home, Bernard is now able to make himself understood, at least concerning his more immediate needs. Speech therapy has been one of the most important aspects of Bernard's training. It seems that he was suffering from some sort of speech defect over and above his general low intelligence. This was recognised by Miss Wallace, when she saw that his comprehension of the spoken word was so much greater than his powers of conversation. The speech therapy which followed has certainly produced great benefits for Bernard. He will never be a great talker, but he is acquiring sufficient speech to give him a considerable degree of independence.

We are told by the Speech Therapy Department that three different factors account for Bernard's difficulties in learning to talk. (1) A very poor ability to remember the nature and order of the sounds which make up a word. He could imitate words correctly immediately after hearing them, but not a minute or two later. (2) An inability to organise, at conversational speed, the complex series of mouth movements necessary to articulate accurately more than four speech sounds in a series. (3) A short span of attention. On the other hand we are also told that Bernard has shown 'a willingness, indeed a determination, to try to speak'.

One of the great difficulties in helping Bernard to talk has been to decide how much effort he is making. At times he appears downright lazy. We have no doubt at all that if left to himself he would have talked only to the extent of making grunts and noises incomprehensible to anyone but himself. It is only because of the effort on our part that he can now make himself understood to strangers. Yet at times he could try so hard to tell us something, that he opened his mouth but nothing came out, and he was in danger of stammering. Indeed, this was the reason why his lessons at the hospital came to an end at the age of fourteen. On many occasions, however, it is far from obvious whether he is trying or not, and one has to make the best judgment one can.

Finally we recount one more episode to stress again the importance of steady encouragement, and also the effect of emotional stress. The episode concerns one of my attempts to make him differentiate between 'Daddy' and 'David'. 'Daddy' comes out very clearly, but 'David' is more difficult, and either sounds like 'Daddy', or perhaps 'Diddi'. One day at tea Bernard was sitting opposite me at the dining-room table, and noticed that David was not present.

'Diddi, no.'

'Who?' I asked.

'Diddi.'

'David,' I said.

'Diddi,' said Bernard, looking cross and turning his head away from me.

'Look at me, and say Day.'

'Day,' said Bernard, looking across at me.

'Right, now say vid.'

'Id.'

'Look at me, bite your lip, and say vid.'

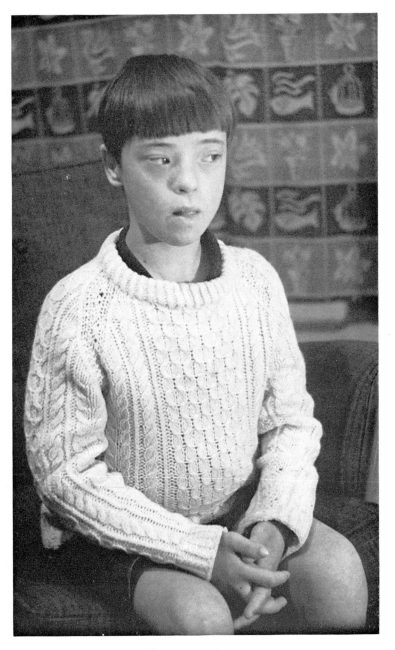

19 Trouble on the way? Bernard nearly 13

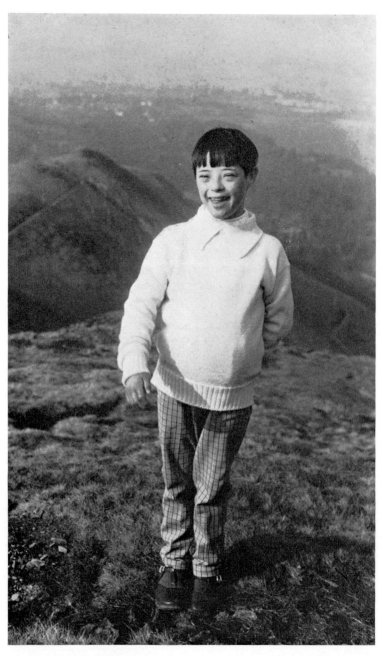

20   On Catbells, Bernard at $13\frac{1}{2}$

'Vid.'

'Now tap it out with your hand, Day-vid.'

Bernard did not listen to the whole word but as I said 'Day', interrupted with his own 'vid'.

'Listen first,' I said, 'then tap it out afterwards, Day-vid.'

This time Bernard did listen. He said 'Day', and then tapped with his hand. He paused again, and we could see a light dawn in his eyes, and he said 'vid'. You could almost see his little brain working.

'Jolly good,' I said, and Bernard beamed.

When David came home from school next day, Bernard was in the kitchen with Eileen and Françoise, our current *au pair*. They all saw David through the window, so Eileen immediately said to Bernard,

'Who's this?'

'Diddi,' said Bernard.

'Daddy is in the lounge,' replied Eileen.

This made Bernard so cross, that he said correctly, 'No, Day-vid.'

Chapter 15

Bernard at Fourteen

We now take a general look at Bernard at about the age of fourteen. He was still very small for his age, being only 4' 6" high, and weighing 5 st. 6 lb. Unlike many mongols he carried no fat, being slight and muscular. Indeed his body was, and is, so supple that a favourite parlour trick is to bring both feet up, and cross his ankles behind his head! In the past, we have often found him asleep in a rather similar jack knife position, with his feet on the pillow beside his head.

Bernard was by now a good walker, although sometimes a reluctant one. It largely depended how interested he was in the matter in hand. He very much liked to walk with me to collect the car after it had been serviced, because there were many interesting things to see at the garage. One day, I had to collect the car when I was short of time, and Bernard asked if he could come. I was rather doubtful at first, but finally said that he could come provided he walked quickly. In the event, he skipped along the pavement, in front of me, at a great rate.

On our holidays, over the years, we have encouraged him in some mild hill-walking, and his powers are quite comparable with those of a normal child of his size. We first took him up the little hill Catbells above Derwent Water when he was 10½ years old. We chose the shortest and easiest way, so that the car made half the height, but Bernard was not at all happy. He paid no attention to where he was putting his feet, got his shoes very wet, and arrived at the top in a rather poor humour (*Plate 15*). Yet on the way back it was obvious that he had not been overtired. He ran down with Maureen, each trying to see who could go the faster. He avoided boggy patches with no trouble, co-operated in walking across the streams, and was obviously enjoying himself. No doubt, too, he was cheered up by the sight of the car in the distance.

The following year, driving along by the side of Derwent Water, we looked across at Catbells. 'Look Bernard, there's Catbells, you went up there last year, wasn't that good?' Bernard's answer was a quite clear 'No more'. However, later in the year, he agreed to be jollied along to the top of Croagh Patrick, standing 2,500 feet above Clew Bay in Ireland.

Bernard's walking ability has steadily improved. When he was nearly thirteen, we took him for a walk through the woods above Grindelwald in Switzerland. As we walked along the path, he and Maureen played hide-and-seek, by climbing off the path into the woods. These woods rose abruptly from the path, but Bernard was able to scramble up the steep slopes with ease. At one time he was seen to place his foot up on to the sloping ground *at the level of his head*, push up from this remarkable position, and then repeat the whole process to gain more height. The following year he joined the whole family in going up Catbells from the Keswick end, that is by the steepest and longest way. He went up very well, made no complaints, and reached the top happily (*Plate 20*). It was also on this holiday that he made the 3-hour walk to Watendlath by Dock Tarn and back, alone with David.

Over the years, Bernard's powers of communication had improved considerably, and now at fourteen he had become much more of a personality. For example, when Bernard was younger he was unable to tell us anything of what went on at school, or on visits to his friends' homes. However, he could now give us some idea of what he had been doing, although he was not always very eager to do so. For example, he was once invited to a party organised by the local branch of the Free Foresters for about a hundred children, of whom about ten were mentally handicapped. When Eileen went to collect Bernard at the end of the party, she found that there had been a film show, and that each child had been given a box of assorted chocolates, a funny hat, an orange and an apple. On their return, we all sat down to supper together.

'Was it a good party, Bernard?' I asked.

'Yes, yes,' replied Bernard brightly, pronouncing the words very clearly.

'What did you do there?'

'Dunno.'

'You don't know?'

'No,' said Bernard, and returned to his supper.

'Bernard!' I said sharply.

Bernard put down his knife and fork, and looked at me somewhat anxiously.

'Now think. You must remember what you did.' Bernard looked desperately at Mummy.

'It's no good looking at me, I wasn't there,' said Eileen. There was a pause, and we could almost hear Bernard thinking.

'Chair,' came triumphantly from Bernard.

'Musical chairs,' translated Eileen.

'Oh yes,' I said. 'Did you win?'

'Yes, er no.'

'And what else did you do?' I asked.

The inquisition was too much for Bernard, he downed his knife and fork and, elbow on table, rested his head in his hand.

'Are you tired?' I asked.

'Yes.'

'Well you had better go to bed.'

Mummy interrupted, 'Aren't you thinking Bernard?'

'Yes,' said Bernard brightly.

'Oh,' I said, 'and have you thought of anything?'

'Apple, orange, chocolate.'

I did not pursue the matter further, but Eileen said, 'There were about a hundred children at the party, and they had a film show. It was very kind of the organisers.'

'Oh,' I said, 'you had a film show, did you?'

'Yes, yes.'

We did not try to find out what the films were about!

Bernard was now an expert at communicating by the art of miming. Indeed, being rather lazy, he preferred to mime even when he should have been talking. The miming was often remarkably clear, at least to the person for whom it was intended. 'Slide', accompanied by waving an arm downwards, was a request for me to pull our screen down and give a show of colour slides. Two pronounced sniffs in the car, one after the other, was a reminder that it was time to buy more petrol. The rather ill-pronounced word 'church', plus both hands being shaken up and down, meant to Eileen 'Can we go and play on Shotover Hill after church?' (The shaking mimed the motion of the car on the rough ground at the top of the hill.)

Besides Bernard getting his meaning across to us, we could also get ours across to him. One day, instead of sitting up at the table, he was drooping down on to his chin and elbows. I became tired of making repeated requests for him to sit up, and said, 'If you don't sit up in future, I am not going to tell you again. You will just get down from the table, and that will be the end of your meal.' This complicated speech was well understood, for he sat up for the rest of the meal, and Eileen noticed him keeping a watchful eye on me.

We have already mentioned that Bernard tended to worry before going away on the annual school holiday. In his last year at school he knew that he was going a full fortnight in advance. Although he seemed to be looking forward to it, he began to twist his handkerchief nervously round and round between his fingers. He knew he would be coming back, but something else was worrying him. For the first time we were able to discuss his fears with him. We asked whether he was going to miss Mummy. This was the trouble. 'Would you like Mummy to come with you?' 'Yes.' 'Would you like Daddy to come with you?' 'No.' This might all sound a rather inconclusive conversation, but afterwards, there was no more twisting of the handkerchief.

Along with his increasing powers of communication, Bernard was at last developing a greater sense of time, and a rather better memory. When he was twelve, we took him on his tenth annual visit to Chapel Farm in the Lake District. The turning where we leave the public road for the final lane to the farm is in a prominent position right by the village school. Therefore, as a test, I stopped the car at the turning and asked Bernard which way to go. To our surprise, he did not know; even though he certainly recognised the farm itself two minutes later. However, a year later there was no doubt that he knew the way.

Other evidence of the improvement in Bernard's memory starts on our summer holiday at Grindelwald, when Bernard went off on an entirely unauthorised haymaking expedition. As we describe this episode later, we need only say here that we were cross with him when he returned. A full six months afterwards, Eileen was discussing with the children where we might go for our next holiday.

'What's wrong with Grindelwald?' asked Andrew.

'No hay Mamma, no hay Mamma,' said Bernard.

'Oh, did you enjoy the haymaking?'

'Yes.'

'It was naughty not to tell anyone.'

'Yes.'

This was the first time that Bernard himself had volunteered the information that he had been haymaking!

Although Bernard's powers of memory are generally quite modest we have often been impressed by how effective they can be on matters which really interest him. Perhaps the best example of all occurred some time ago. Bernard has always been very interested in mechanical devices, and took a close interest in our car. If Eileen went along for any distance in third gear instead of top, Bernard was sure to point to the gear change lever, and order 'Down'. Just before Christmas when Bernard was ten, he and Eileen went by car to collect Granny to stay with us for the holiday. I had previously put a large sheet of cardboard in front of part of the radiator, to help the engine warm up more quickly. The weather was warm, and when Eileen stopped at her brother's house on the way home, the car was enveloped in clouds of steam. Eileen and her nephew opened the bonnet and saw steam issuing from the radiator, so they left the car to cool off, and then refilled the radiator. Eileen, Bernard and Granny proceeded on their way, but soon the water temperature had again risen above boiling, so Eileen stopped at a garage, to see more steam rising from the radiator. As the garage attendant poured water into the radiator, he saw the cardboard and remarked 'Well, what do you expect, having this in front of the radiator? Quite unnecessary!' The cardboard was then removed.

The next part of this story occurs at Christmas *two years* later. The conditions were similar, it had been very cold in mid-December, but had turned mild just before Christmas. Bernard had seen me put the usual piece of cardboard into position in front of the radiator. As Eileen drove out of Henley, on her way to collect Granny, Bernard said 'Shoosh', and flung his arms up in the air. Eileen immediately looked at the water temperature, and saw that it was near boiling. 'Thank you, Bernard,' she said, and removed the cardboard at the first opportunity. As one might expect, Bernard was very pleased with himself, and had to be given a great big kiss. This was a feat of memory far beyond his usual performance, stimulated by his intense interest in motor cars.

As Bernard's powers of communication and memory improved, he became proficient in bringing verbal messages home from school. He might come to Eileen, with her purse in his hand, and say 'Money—lunch'. Eileen had forgotten to give him his lunch money on Monday, and it was now Thursday. Eileen would put the money into an envelope, and place it on the hall stand. Then without any reminder, he would collect it on Friday morning, and take it off to school.

Besides a sense of time past, or memory, Bernard had now also acquired some sense of time future. In the past, when he knew that he was going away on a family holiday, he would get out a suitcase several days before we were ready to leave, and pack it with his clothes. Eileen would then have to explain that we were not going for a few days, and unpack the case to retrieve the clothes that he would need in the meantime. Explanations had little effect on Bernard, for as like as not he would repack the case the following night. By now, however, we were able to say to him one Monday that he broke up for his summer holidays on the coming Friday, and he understood what was meant. (This success was the result of Eileen spending several hours with Bernard and a calendar.)

By now Bernard could do many useful jobs about the house, and on occasion he was eager to be helpful. Once, when Eileen could not find a saucepan she needed for cooking, Bernard knew where it was and produced it.

'Thank you, Bernard, that was good of you.'

'Hurrah, good me,' says Bernard. And that was the first time he had ever said 'hurrah'.

Earlier that year I was out of the house and Eileen had unexpectedly to visit a friend on urgent business. She put the kettle on for tea and prepared most of the supper. David was about the house, but Maureen was left in charge of the domestic arrangements. Neither I nor Eileen were in for tea or supper. The next morning Eileen thanked Maureen for doing all the domestic chores, and was told that Bernard had helped all the time. He had laid the table for tea and supper, he had washed up the tea things, and some of the cooking pots. Eileen thanked him and he looked very pleased.

Helpful as he could be, Bernard was also sufficient of a normal child to know when to vanish, for example when he saw that supper was almost cooked, and that it was time to lay the table. David and Andrew learned this one years ago! Bernard was also capable of helping Eileen to make the beds, but sometimes he only began to co-operate as I walked into the bedroom. On the other hand, if Bernard thought there was a possibility of a ride in the car, he could be very good and helpful indeed.

Life with Bernard has always been enlivened by the various odd happenings which take place about the house. There was a period when we put up our hand to pull the chain on the high water tank of the W.C., only to find nothing there. The handle and chain were then found either on the top of the tank or inside it. We never knew for certain who was responsible, but in our mind's eye, we all saw Bernard pulling the chain, giving the handle a skilful flick skywards, and then giving a great chuckle as it landed in the tank. Be that as it may, we complained to him, and eventually the chain was left in peace.

Bernard had now a quite well-developed sense of right and wrong, but at times remarkably little guile. On one occasion I happened to be standing in one corner of our bedroom looking at some books. While I was there, Bernard came in with the carpet sweeper, without seeing me. He is not really supposed to use the sweeper unless someone knows what he is doing, and he is certainly not allowed to try to unscrew the handle. Fortunately the handle is fixed in such a way that, although it will rotate, it does not unscrew. I watched Bernard for quite a time as he twisted the handle round and round. Suddenly he looked up and saw me. His face fell. 'Oh Dadda!' he said, picked up the sweeper, and disappeared.

Another example of Bernard's dim optimism showed up when I returned home one day to find Bernard alone on the pavement outside the house, where he had no business to be. Trusting that I had not seen him, he ran quickly back to the house, and in at the back door. The front door was then opened by a smiling, and presumably good, Bernard welcoming Daddy home. Another day we noticed a small dent in the wall of the lounge; we did not know who was responsible, but started asking questions. 'You know where it is, don't you Bernard?' said Mummy. 'Naw.' 'Well, show us where it is,' said Eileen, 'show David the hole in the wall.' Bernard went straight to the wall and showed David the hole.

Bernard's behaviour had improved over the years, and his temper tantrums had gradually died away. However, they had not disappeared completely, and a typical episode occurred when Eileen's mother and another visitor were having tea with her. As they all sat down, Eileen noticed that Bernard's hands were very dirty. 'Bernard your hands are filthy. Go and wash them.' 'No,' he shouted back. Having two guests for tea, Eileen did not insist, but thought, 'He's got away with that.' However, after a pause, he got down from his chair, stamped out from the dining room into the kitchen, and slammed the door. A few minutes later, he stamped back, slamming the door on his way, and with some noise regained his seat. His sleeves were pushed up, and his hands were clean. No comment was made, although Granny almost said 'Oh, so you've washed your hands,' but she thought (correctly) that it would be better to say nothing.

On another occasion, Bernard had been naughty at church one evening, but had eventually calmed down and told Eileen how sorry he was. As it happened, I was not home for supper, and Bernard took one look at the shepherd's pie and screamed 'No'.

'I thought you were sorry for being naughty,' said Eileen.

'No,' was the reply.

'Any more and you will go off to bed.'

At that he started to eat his supper, and then asked for a second helping. Something went wrong about that, Eileen is not sure what and he grabbed at his glass of water and drank the whole large tumbler in one gulp. The water immediately took effect, and supper was finished in peace with Bernard the picture of misery giving out the occasional burp. As this was now one of his worse days, we see that his behaviour had improved very substantially since the tantrums described in chapter 11.

One of Bernard's most endearing traits is his sense of humour. Anything that is obviously funny is much appreciated. He loves the slapstick comedy and custard pie scenes at the pantomime. He appreciates the humour of many everyday situations. Maureen was given a weight-driven clock for Christmas, and she and Bernard took it in turns to wind it up. One day Bernard went up to Eileen with a sweet little smile, and said:

'Mummy, clock, clock.'

'Oh yes, let's do it, is it your turn?'

'Yes,' so he and Eileen wound the clock. As they finished it seemed to Eileen that Bernard was looking rather smug.

'Was it really your turn Bernard?'

'No Maw, Maw,' said the naughty Bernard with a great grin all over his face.

Bernard often likes hiding David's pyjamas in his (Bernard's) bed. Actually, Bernard misses the best of this joke, for he then goes to bed himself, and is sound asleep when David arrives. David now knows where to look for the pyjamas, and untucks the bottom of Bernard's bed without disturbing him.

One of Bernard's favourite ploys when I was away, was playing at being Daddy. On one occasion, he remained upstairs until break-fast was ready, and would not come down until Eileen had called 'Daddy, breakfast ready'. (She usually calls 'John', but refused to humour Bernard to this extent.) Once down, he sat in my place at table and made a great show of propping up the newspaper against the milk jug. Actually the newspaper was upside down, but this did not matter. Usually I get my own breakfast from the kitchen, but he waved an imperious arm at Françoise and Eileen for them to get his breakfast. Françoise was too amused to do anything, as she had not seen these antics before. So Eileen got his breakfast. He ate this, still pretending to be me, turning the paper over, opening it, folding it, and propping it against the milk jug. Next morning, the same pantomime was repeated, but this time the rest of the family made a great point of wanting the milk jug. He was rather put out by this, and kept saying 'Me, Daddy'. He saw that everyone was highly amused, and thoroughly enjoyed his joke.

When I was away from home a few months later, the same performance was repeated, but with a variant. He had obviously been watching me more closely, for when he had finished his bacon and started on his toast, he moved his chair back a little from the table, turned slightly, and crossed one leg over the other. He then held the paper in one hand, while he ate his toast with the other. Françoise was in fits of laughter at this very good imitation of Daddy, but Bernard said sharply, 'No laugh', and solemnly continued his breakfast.

Bernard now began to acquire a capacity for independent action. When we were on holiday at Grindelwald, our chalet was next door to a dairy. We would send Bernard down with the money for the milk, and he would come back with the milk and the change. Similar operations were more difficult at home, because our house is cut off from the shops by busy roads. Even so, Eileen could take him to the hairdresser in the car, give him the money, and send him into the shop by himself. He eventually emerged with his hair duly cut. On other occasions, Eileen wrote on a piece of paper what she wanted, and sent Bernard into the butcher by himself. He managed to buy the meat, collect the change, and bring them out to her.

All through the years, Bernard had been making steady progress, yet it was necessary to view this progress with a patient eye, for compared with that of normal children it is pretty slow progress. It is important to accept a mentally handicapped child as he is, and not be anxious to change him into someone different. We thought that we ourselves had both come to accept this, but a series of episodes caused us to think again.

During our holiday at Grindelwald Bernard was taken for a ride by his friends at the dairy next door. As he did not tell anyone that he was going, no one knew where he was for about half an hour, until he came back. I took a poor view of this, for I thought he was old enough to have told us. However, I found myself in a minority of one. It was not really Bernard's fault, his friends in the car should have made sure that we knew. Eileen was impressed that Bernard had said, very contritely, that he was sorry, and that he understood that he should not have gone. I remained at heart unconvinced by all this, but went along with Eileen's view that he was, in fact, becoming more mature.

Our faith in Bernard was not altogether justified. During the next two weeks of the holiday he again went absent without leave on two occasions. The first time he fortunately ran into David in the village, and was brought back home. The second time he went off with two of the neighbouring farmers, on their tractor, to go hay-making. Eileen and I were out at the time, and Manuela (our *au pair* from Portugal) had no idea where he was. As he was away for most of the afternoon, she eventually went down and reported his loss to the police. At this stage he came back. This episode did not seem to me an example of very mature behaviour, but I was assured that it was really the fault of the farmers for taking him.

When we returned home, there were further signs, if one chose to look, that all was not quite well. Eileen found that Bernard was being particularly difficult at times; he was awkward when buying clothes and not so good in church. One day she told him not to open a can of fruit for lunch, and he immediately opened it. He impressed his attention on me by a series of fiddlings about the house. Opening a new book of postage stamps I found that all the stamps had been torn out, and then replaced in position. One day he pushed over the main electricity switch. Another day we had to retrieve most of our garden tools from the front gardens of various houses anything up to 100 yards away.

The climax came one morning when we found that someone had played with the coke stove that heats the water, and had displaced the bottom grid that holds the fire in position. It looked as if Master Bernard had been in sight of moving a can of red hot ash about the house. At this stage, I put my foot down, and said we were not going to have Bernard wandering round the house in the early mornings, completely irresponsible, fiddling with every tap and device he could lay his hands on. He was therefore brought down from the bedroom where he slept with Andrew and David, and put by himself in the nursery, whose door was then hooked up so that it would not open more than a couple of inches. He did not like this change at all, but was told that he could only go back upstairs after he had shown that he could behave himself properly for a few days. In fact, his behaviour improved immediately, and after about a fortnight he was back in his normal bedroom. It was then a matter of several months before he got into any other major scrape.

There is a moral to this last story. Eileen and I both thought that we took a fairly objective view of Bernard. Yet Eileen had been over-optimistic about Bernard's progress and degree of responsibility, and had taken this view right up until the episode of the stove. She was then really quite upset, to her surprise and mine, when it became all too plain that progress was not as fast as she had thought. Deep instincts tend to make us push our children forward, but they are not always very helpful or useful.

Chapter 16

Bernard Today

Bernard is now seventeen. He is still very small for his age being only 5' 1" tall. His speech and vocabulary have improved, although strangers still have difficulty in understanding him at first. His powers of comprehension are better and he can count up to ten, and reel off the days of the week. Last, but by no means least, his behaviour has steadily improved; he still argues a great deal, but very seldom throws a tantrum in his old manner.

Bernard can now wash and dress himself reliably, although Eileen sometimes has rather an argument to get him started on these operations. He can tie a granny knot but not a bow, and finds buttons difficult, and is therefore quite content for mum to attend to his shoe laces and ties. Indeed, one of his most characteristic expressions when his laces need tying is to go up to Eileen, show her his hands, grin, and say 'Can't do'. One day he even tried an alternative approach by going up to Dominique, our *au pair*, showing her his laces and saying 'Slave'!

In the house Bernard can make a good job of sweeping the floor, washing up, making beds and ironing. He can lay the table for a meal, prepare coffee and bring it in on a tray, and act as a waiter. If I am working in the garden, I can ask him for a tool, and he will bring it from the house. He will also make a good job of sweeping up leaves, putting them into a barrow, and taking them to a dump. If I am working on the car, and drop a nut, he will probably be the first to find it. He can serve Mass. He can milk a cow by hand, but rather blotted his copy book one day at Chapel Farm one Easter, when he was found with a third of a bucket of milk which he had just taken from a cow in the middle of the afternoon.

It is noticeable that Bernard has now begun to persevere at a task even if it does not go right the first time. A few months ago, I saw him filling a bowl of water at the wash basin in the bathroom. When full, the bowl was quite heavy, and difficult to remove from the basin without spilling some of the water. Bernard did not know that I was watching, and when his first attempt failed, he put the bowl back in the basin, and gave a little dance of rage. He then made another attempt, which again failed, and was followed by another little dance. However, at the third attempt the bowl was safely removed without losing any water.

A most important event for Bernard came about a year ago, when he seemed to have taken in everything the school could offer him, and was getting a bit bored. He was therefore transferred to the Industrial Training Unit which he now attends daily. When Bernard was born, the only provision for the mentally handicapped of all ages were the so-called occupation centres, where they remained for their whole life. When we first heard of these centres they sounded unattractive. We gained the impression that the work done by the older people was very simple, very routine and very dull. At the time, however, we saw no point in making further enquiries. Today, the position is rather different. It is now official government policy to provide satisfying 'permanent daily occupation for mentally handicapped adults who are not able to work in open or sheltered employment'. The standards of provision of such work centres is still variable across the country, but we are fortunate in having a very good one in Oxford.

The work centre which Bernard attends is called an Industrial Training Unit, or ITU. The ITU is situated in an attractive and modern building, in a pleasant part of the city. The main workshop is light and airy with a spacious layout, but quite similar in appearance to what one might find in any ordinary factory. At one end is a spacious loading bay for lorries to bring in and carry away the work. This main workshop is supported by a whole range of ancillary rooms, including two smaller workrooms where a closer watch may be kept on new entrants. There is also a room with equipment for giving further training in domestic subjects and in more general topics. By far the largest of the ancillary buildings is the hall which serves as an assembly area, as the dining room at lunch-time, and as a meeting place during the morning and afternoon breaks. Finally, there is a kitchen to cook the lunch, cloakrooms, and offices. At present there is room in the workshops for 60 people, but all the services and facilities in the ancillary rooms are designed for 120 people, so that the workshop may be extended in the future to accommodate this larger number.

Most of the young people coming to the ITU will probably never be able to take a normal job. On the other hand, nearly all of them will be capable of useful and interesting work, if it can be provided in a sheltered environment. Some will probably be capable of working in the normal community after a further period of training. The unit therefore aims to provide interesting and stimulating work for all its members, in such a way that those who are capable may eventually progress into an ordinary job. It is also the aim of the unit to train the adults to take their part, to a greater or lesser extent, in all aspects of normal social life. Hence, the routine in the unit is planned to be closely parallel to life outside.

As we have said, the building itself has been designed to resemble a modern factory, and the work is done under conditions quite similar to those in ordinary workshops. The trainees work a 5-day week, from 9.15 a.m. to 4.15 p.m. each day, travel from their homes unescorted in a special coach, and clock in on arrival. Each trainee is paid a small wage, which is worked out on a scale which takes account not only of his output for the week, but also of his effort, so that a severely handicapped person working to his full capacity is not penalised.

The unit has been fortunate in having good friends in the adjacent motor car works, who have given a great deal of help in setting up the unit and in finding suitable work. The machines used by the trainees include drilling machines, fly presses, a sanding machine, a circular saw, and a spot welder, all carefully provided with safety guards so that no one gets hurt. A wide variety of work is done for many different outside firms. These jobs include assembling sets of motor car components, packing glove boxes, assembling water pump kits, making swabs and plastic bibs, stitching hand guards, sorting plastics, cutting paper, drilling castors, etc. These products are just as good, or perhaps even better, than those produced in a normal factory. In assembling sets of components, the various items are placed in holes in a jig to ensure that nothing is overlooked. The final job is then checked by another trainee, who will note any omissions. We are told that the trainees have the reputation of being a very reliable set of workers.

Another feature of the ITU is the continuation of the social training which was given to the children all the time they were attending school. As before, this training is not directed towards book learning, but to those skills which are most helpful in every-day life, such as the recognition of simple key words like 'stop', 'push', 'W.C.', 'danger' and 'private'. At lunch-times, the trainees pick up their meals in cafeteria fashion then sit at tables for four, selecting their own places with their friends. A vending machine for hot drinks gives them experience in using coin-operated mach-ines. The girls are taught to care for their personal appearance, lessons are given in hairdressing and they have the use of a helmet dryer.

From what we have said, it is clear that the name 'Industrial Training Unit' does not give an altogether exact description of the unit. Its main function is to provide a workshop where the handi-capped can perform real and useful tasks in a sheltered environ-ment. To do this work, the handicapped must of course be trained, hence the name of the unit. Even so, we have heard it said that, to get even better results one should separate the two functions of training and providing sheltered workshops. Be that as it may, when we first visited the ITU two or three years before Bernard went there, we were immediately struck by the alert and interested way in which the majority of the trainees approach their work. Since then, we have always been impressed by the happy atmosphere, which is set by the manager and his staff, and by the other city officials responsible for the unit.

Bernard settled into the ITU with very little disturbance, so far as we could discern from his behaviour at home. The daily routine of catching the coach outside our house in the morning and coming back in the afternoon was the same as for school. His hours away from home were slightly longer but this did not seem to worry him. Once or twice he asked when he would be going back to his old school (we were then calling the ITU his new school to help the transition), but he went off each morning with no more fuss than usual. He was certainly very pleased with himself when he brought home his first pay packet, and proudly showed it to every member of the family.

We gather that Bernard is developing into a reliable worker although it is only recently that we have discovered what he actually does. Initially he was extremely reluctant to tell us any-thing about his day at the unit. 'Don't know', was the standard reply for nearly a year. Then one evening at supper he said, with-

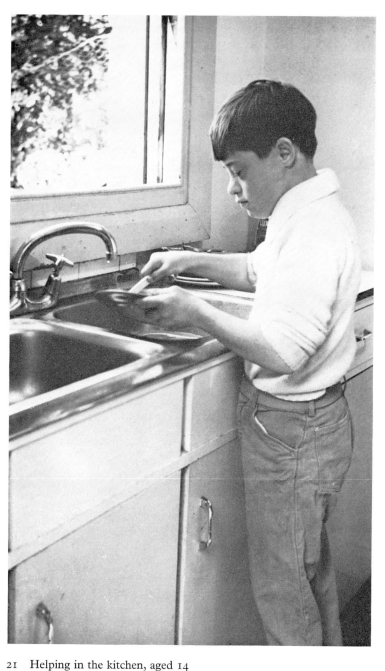

21 Helping in the kitchen, aged 14

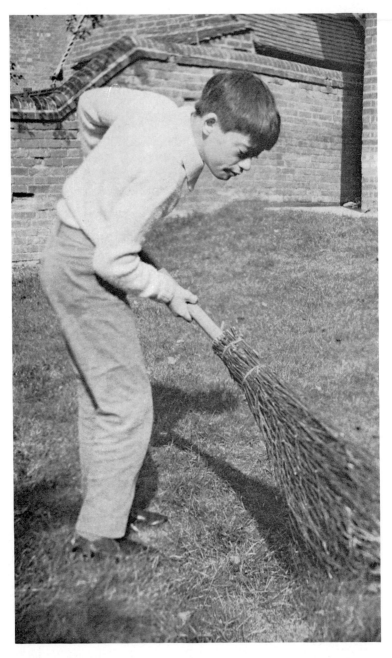

22 Working in the garden, aged 14

out any questioning from us, 'Sausages school', and a few months later he said 'Sellotape box', and mimed how to Sellotape a box. From time to time we also hear of some of his friends, but not very much, and he has told us when some of them from school have joined him at the ITU.

Recently some friends of ours were shown round the unit and they saw Bernard at work before he saw them and recognised them. These friends have known Bernard for many years and they told us how impressed they were by his calm attitude at work. We gather from the manager of the unit, Mr Price, that he can 'have his days', but all in all there is the feeling that he is growing up and becoming better behaved. No doubt all this is helped by the knowledge he now has that if he does not work properly he does not receive so much money.

An annual week's holiday for the trainees is organised jointly by the ITU and the Oxford branch of the National Association for Mentally Handicapped Children. It takes the form of a camp run by volunteers at the city's outdoor-pursuit centre in Wales. Bernard went for the first time when he was sixteen; he had just come home from a family holiday but was very pleased to be going away by himself. Unlike the school holidays when he was younger he did not worry; he did not wring his handkerchief and he did not pack his bag every evening during the preceding week, and did not want to pack his entire wardrobe. He went off happily and returned happily and told us of the highlights of the week. It was obvious that he had thoroughly enjoyed himself and he is eagerly looking forward to the next instalment.

Another important change for Bernard occurred about eighteen months ago, when Eileen's mother came to live with us. Granny was then eighty-four, and although in quite good general health, was finding it difficult to get about and look after herself in her own home. She now lives with us in her own bed-sitting room, which is large enough to accommodate her television set (the only one in the house) and all the family who wish to watch it. Bernard is very fond of Granny and does a great deal to help look after her; he is also very fond of watching her television set. In fact these two aspects of his life with Granny are almost impossible to separate!

When Bernard is at home, he nearly always takes Granny her meals. He brings in her early morning cup of tea, tidies her pillows, gives her her glasses, and then waits with her until it is time to catch the bus. He keeps the room tidy, waters the plants, keeps her jug of water full, pours out her lemon squash, and sees that she has her apples and sweets. On Sundays he takes her out for her little afternoon walk, much to her amusement as he thinks she is very slow, and often tries to hurry her along so as to get back to the television.

Bernard is a great companion for Granny because they both like the same sort of television programmes: cowboys, funnies and thrillers. As a result he is seldom in the kitchen with Mummy, and no longer available to lay the table. In fact the only time in the evening that he is seen in the kitchen is during the news. Hopefully, he then wants supper immediately so as to avoid missing the next programme, and when supper is eventually finished he is always the first to disappear back to the telly. For really important programmes like 'Laurel and Hardy' and 'The Virginian' he is allowed to have his supper with Granny.

One considerable use of the television is in persuading Bernard to behave himself properly. Even the mention of not watching television generally produces a very marked improvement in his manner. As for not being allowed to watch for a week, that is a very severe punishment indeed. Yet there is a difficulty over this type of punishment. Bernard generally finds something else to do, but Granny finds that she misses Bernard. Bernard has now become aware of this, and if banned from the television says to Eileen, 'Poor Granny—no me.'

For her part, Granny does a great deal to help Bernard. After he has taken Granny her early morning cup of tea, he produces the *Radio Times* so she can tell him what is on television that evening. However, Bernard has first to spell out the appropriate day of the week, and can now pronounce them all and spell out d-a-y. He can also work out how many days remain before his favourite programme. Other lessons from Granny have taught him to count reliably up to ten, and his proficiency was very noticeable last Christmas when he was counting the pound notes he had received as presents. Granny also reads his library books to him when they are not both watching telly. She has also been trying to teach Bernard to read, by pronouncing the names of words written out on cards, and he can now recognise words such as Bernard Wilks, danger, Monday, Tuesday, etc.

Granny also helps Bernard with his speech. His vocabulary is steadily increasing, although he still speaks mainly with nouns together with adverbs and conjunctions, never in sentences. He tries to say more and more words, but his diction remains indistinct, and he tends to shout if not understood the first time. Granny has been coaching him to say 'Bernard Wilks', followed by our address, sufficiently distinctly that a stranger could understand. She has her ups and downs with this tuition. Sometimes he objects strongly and shouts at her, then she responds with 'No television if you shout'. Sometimes this has an effect, at other times Eileen has to sort out the commotion with the result that Bernard has to be withdrawn from all television for the rest of the evening. Then there are *two* unhappy members of the family, and we find that Granny is being punished more than Bernard!

As a result of this mutual aid, Bernard and Granny have come to share a considerable rapport. On one occasion recently Eileen had to see to Granny in the morning because Bernard had hurt his hand. As Granny struggled to sit up in bed, she said rather plaintively to Eileen, 'Oh dear, I can't sit up any more', and sank back on the pillows. Eileen was rather surprised because usually she finds Granny sitting up very well of a morning. Granny then continued even more plaintively, 'I'll soon not be able to sit up in bed at all'. At this moment Bernard came into the room; he took one look at Granny and promptly said, 'Granny, UP'. To Eileen's astonishment Granny promptly struggled a little and sat up. 'See, Granny', said Bernard. Eileen left the two of them together.

Over the years Bernard has become more independent and more capable of doing things by himself. However, his progress is rather uncertain, and he is always ready to slide back into bad habits. This point is illustrated very well by his table manners. When he is in good form, his behaviour would pass muster on any occasion, and we could take him anywhere without embarrassment. However, this behaviour does not follow invariably day by day at home. Left to himself he tends to slump lower and lower in his chair, his face comes nearer and nearer to his plate, and his nose almost touches his food. He then has to be told to sit up and eat properly, which he then does, with a varying amount of fuss, depending on who asked him.

We wish to encourage him to become independent, but it is a slow process. For example, he is now able to wait for the coach in the morning on the pavement outside our house by himself, but considerable supervision of this exercise is still needed. First of all, he has to be told not once, but several times, that it is time to go out. The pavement is wide outside our house, so that he can safely stand by the garden wall away from the traffic. We must, however, keep an eye on him to make sure that he is not doing either a song or a dance all by himself on the pavement. This only happens occasionally, but it must make a rather odd impression on any passer-by. Finally, we must be sure that he is on the pavement when the bus arrives, and not wandering back to the front door.

Last winter when the weather became colder, Bernard began to complain when the bus was a few minutes late, even though he was well wrapped up against the cold. On one occasion, after waiting outside for fifteen minutes, Bernard came back to the front door and shouted through the letter-box 'No bus. Cold'. Eileen opened the front door and he came in looking cold. She said 'But the bus will be here in a minute, you must go out to wait for it. It will not stop if you are not on the pavement.' Bernard was by then warming himself at the heater in the hall and said 'No'. Eileen repeated 'Go on out'. 'No'. At that moment Eileen saw the coach go by without stopping, and told Bernard, who went out like a flash to see it disappearing down the road. He was momentarily disconcerted, but brightened up and said 'Car'. Meanwhile I had appeared, having heard the entire proceedings, and I said 'No car, you heard Mummy tell you to go out and wait, and you refused, you will have to stay at home for the day. And you will not spend the day with Granny watching television. You will not go into Granny's room until the usual time this evening.' This was the end, Bernard's face screwed up and tears trickled down his cheeks.

Eileen, left to herself, would have taken him to the ITU and Bernard would have seen even less reason to wait outside in future. As it is, he has now got the message that if he wants to go to the ITU, he must put up with the normal day-to-day discomforts of all of us who have to wait for a bus on a cold morning. At any event, he has not returned from the pavement since. Moreover he is at last realising that there are sound reasons for behaving in a certain way, and not always choosing the immediately easiest or pleasant line of action. He is in fact slowly growing up.

Another way in which he is growing up is that his upper lip is showing considerable sign of a moustache and his genitals have developed, 'Me big boy now'. However, apart from this there are not many other changes. He has always been more demonstrably affectionate towards people, both family, friends, and even mere acquaintances, than our other children. This is a well-known characteristic of mongols and we have tried to restrain him from the too boisterous embrace and the too affectionate kiss. This became more necessary as he grew older, and is still necessary today. From time to time, Eileen has to discourage him from turning his good-night kiss to her into a scene from the telly. We have also persuaded him to wear a dressing gown when he goes wandering round the house with not much on.

Chapter 17

Helping Parents

This account of Bernard is a personal story, which tells the tale of one particular family with one particular handicapped child. We have been helped in bringing up Bernard both by our own situation and by the quality of the various services provided by the local authorities. We have had advantages not open to everyone, but the parents of any mentally handicapped child find themselves faced by the same kinds of problems. Therefore we now look back on the ways in which we were helped, to show how other parents might be helped in the future.

One of the most important factors in bringing up Bernard has been that Eileen was engaged in work at the laboratory; this had important consequences. First of all, we could afford to have an *au pair* girl to work about the house and help look after the children. We have described the labour involved in dealing with all the extra day-to-day chores of bringing up a handicapped child. We have mentioned the labour and work involved in training Bernard to eat properly, in toilet training, and in dealing with his tantrums. Other parents would include other items, perhaps the effort to contain wandering around the house, and the consequent loss of sleep. The presence of the *au pair* made it possible for Eileen to give the normal necessary attention to the other children, particularly in their younger days. The *au pair* looked after Bernard while Eileen helped the other children with their homework, reading, and other activities. We do not see how we could have been fair to the other children without this extra pair of hands.

There is a clear case for providing some form of domestic assistance for the parents of mentally handicapped children, similar perhaps to schemes for aiding the physically handicapped. For example, a visitor who could attend to the handicapped child each afternoon when the other children returned from school, would help the whole family. Then again some parents of handicapped children find it very difficult to get away from the home for any social life of their own, so voluntary help in baby-sitting arrangements could be very valuable. Also, for most parents, the holidays provided for the children by the school and the ITU are doubly valuable, as besides giving the children a change they also permit the parents to relax for a while.

Even apparently trivial ways of helping parents may be very important. As we live on a main road, the school bus and the ITU bus pass our house every morning, and pick up Bernard straight from the door, and return him in the evening. However, when Bernard first started school, Eileen had to take him a mile down the road to wait for the bus every morning, and then collect him again every evening. These trips were often troublesome, as at that time Bernard tended to run away if given any opportunity. The bus was sometimes ten or fifteen minutes late, and it seemed that this happened most frequently on cold and wet mornings. I myself remember waiting to collect Bernard off the bus one cold December evening for over an hour, because no one had remembered to tell the parents that the children were having a Christmas party and would be late. The business of having to take a child to and from the bus, for a distance of up to a mile away, every day, in all weathers, can be extremely trying. Indeed, to a mother with other children, this transport problem might well be an important factor in convincing her that she can no longer look after the child at home.

Nursery schools can provide valuable training for the child, and at the same time give needed relief to the mother. Bernard's brothers, David and Andrew, both went to a private nursery school from the age of two, where they could play each morning, and mix with other children. Bernard developed so slowly, that he was $4\frac{1}{2}$ years before he reached the same stage as David and Andrew at the age of two. We then made enquiries, and learnt that he could start immediately at the Mabel Prichard School, so the question of sending him to a nursery school never arose. However, if a handicapped child were more forward physically than Bernard, it might be very desirable for him to attend a nursery school, both for his own benefit and to help his mother.

Another important consequence of Eileen working at the labora-

tory was that for a large part of the day she left the house and concentrated her thoughts on matters other than Bernard. Eileen was
fortunate in having this work to occupy her attention, but for a
woman burdened with a handicapped child all the time the position
could be very different. One recalls Balzac's description of Eugénie
Grandet waiting over the years for her absent lover.

> In every situation a woman is bound to suffer in many ways
> that a man does not, and to feel her troubles more acutely
> than he can; for a man's vigour and energy is constantly
> brought into play; he acts and thinks, comes and goes, busies
> himself in the present, and looks to the future for consolation.
> . . . But a woman cannot help herself—hers is a passive part;
> she is left face to face with her trouble, and has nothing to
> divert her mind from it; she sounds the depths of the abyss
> of sorrow, and its dark places are filled with her prayers and
> tears.

In addition to the help of the *au pair* girl and Eileen's outside
interests, we have also been very fortunate in the support of our
other three children. We hope that it is clear from what we have
written above that all three of them are very fond of Bernard,
treat him as one of themselves, and do a great deal to look after
him. Of course, the larger the family, the easier does this mutual
help become; for example, we have described how Bernard has
helped to look after Granny. An essential feature of our situation
was that our family unit consisted for most of the time of seven
people; ourselves, our four children, and the *au pair* girl. With
such a group it is possible to absorb one retarded or handicapped
member, without excessive work or dislocation of the activities of
the whole group.

Even with these advantages, all has not been plain sailing for us.
The position would be much more difficult if, for example, the
family consisted of mother, father and one retarded child. Left to
itself, without any assistance, such a family is hardly a viable
unit. Then again, if the child grows into a large strong boy with
an urge to wander, he will provide a very difficult problem for his
parents. Because Bernard has remained at home, it does not follow
that it is always possible for a child to remain at home. One cannot
generalise from our experience with Bernard to the best way of
bringing up mongol and handicapped children with quite different
personalities and backgrounds.

136

It is, however, almost certainly true that all parents will find it difficult at first to accept the child as he is. We take it as natural that parents should be proud of a new baby who is healthy, blooming and intelligent. Yet there is clearly an inbuilt antithesis between a ready willingness to accept a handicapped child and the desire of parents to take a pride in their children, to help them forward, and to see them 'succeed'. There is also another and more subtle antithesis, which cannot be resolved without some sense of strain. Bernard can now behave very reasonably, and has some power of speech, but this has only come about as the result of much training both at home and at school. As we have described many times in the previous chapters, Bernard's behaviour often appeared to us to be either downright lazy or downright naughty. It was then most necessary for us not to accept his performance, but to ask him to do better. On innumerable occasions one has to decide whether the reason for a poor performance is because the child is not trying, or because the task is too hard for him. These decisions will often be very difficult for the parents.

As we have already mentioned, an important way in which all parents gain help in bringing up their children is by talking with other parents. The exchange of experiences and information about ordinary children comes very naturally between friends and neighbours, but is more difficult for parents of handicapped children. The children at Bernard's school come from an area several miles across, so special efforts have to be made if parents are to meet. Hence the parent-teacher associations of the local school plays a particularly important role in bringing parents together, besides allowing them to meet their children's teachers. Associations such as the National Association for Mentally Handicapped Children and the Catholic Handicapped Children's Fellowship also provide opportunities for parents to get together both with and without their children.

Meetings like the above can lead on to less formal ones, like the day to day casual encounters when normal children are discussed. Some time ago, a group of Eileen's friends whom she knew through the PTA and by taking Bernard's friends home from his birthday parties, organised a series of coffee mornings or lunches or coffee evenings. These meetings, just for the mothers, served as a form of group therapy. Everyone talked freely about their problems and they all found relief in the discovery that problems they thought were peculiar to themselves, were in fact common to others.

We have been fortunate in the various health and local authority services provided for Bernard but we know that not all parents have been equally fortunate. Schools, training units and hostel facilities often fall far below the standards we have described in Oxford.

Bernard has always received good medical attention, but other children sometimes fare differently. Although mentally handicapped children often require better medical attention than the average, they may receive much *worse*. Many doctors and consultants treat the mentally handicapped with care and sympathy, but a sizeable number seem to take the view that if you are mentally handicapped there is not much need to trouble about your physical ailments. We know of a doctor who refused to prescribe spectacles for a young boy suffering from astigmatism, and of another who dealt with a child with runny eyes by remarking 'Oh, they do'. There is sometimes a reluctance to provide hearing aids for deaf children, presumably on the assumption that it is a waste of time and money to make provision for the mentally handicapped. The school doctor system has not always worked as efficiently for handicapped as for normal children, and the school dentist is sometimes non-existent.

Bernard's speech has improved enormously as a result of speech therapy, but he was very fortunate to receive these lessons. Generally, speech therapy departments do not have time to do much for children like Bernard. This is largely because there is a shortage of trained speech therapists, but there is also another influence at work. It seems that many speech therapists take the same sort of view of the mentally handicapped as those doctors who refuse to provide spectacles and hearing aids. A standard current textbook on speech therapy says, 'If the mental deficiency is extreme, one can scarcely consider seriously giving speech therapy with the expectation of significant results'. Our experience with Bernard is quite different. Speech therapy has enabled Bernard to say a range of simple words, so that he can make himself understood to strangers, at least to some extent. All this was achieved without making excessive demands on the speech therapists. Clearly there is a limit to the time which can be spent giving Bernard speech therapy. Even after a lifetime's course, we are sure that he would still require more therapy before he could speak properly. Yet we are equally sure that it is very important to help the handicapped child to make a small advance, which may greatly benefit him, as in the case of Bernard.

We described in chapter 3 the excellent advice that we received from many quarters after Bernard was born. The advice we received was very extensive. We had the benefit of discussions with our own general practitioner, with a consulting paediatrician, with our friend Keith Lovell, another paediatrician, with Eileen's cousin, a consulting neurologist, with the headmaster of the ESN School, with three sets of parents, with two priests, and with friends who had experience of mental handicap. This is a long list, but we were certainly grateful to have had the opportunity of talking to so many people. As a result, we accepted the diagnosis, and obtained a very adequate picture of how Bernard would grow up, and what action was necessary in the immediate future. It is essential that parents of handicapped children receive this type of advice from the earliest moment, and that this should be given by people with a full understanding of the problems including the genetic aspects mentioned in chapter 4. It is also very important that they are soon given the opportunity to meet parents of children similar to their own.

In the end, however, the most important interactions are those between the parents and the rest of the community. We have already referred to the difficulty that parents may have in coming to accept a handicapped child as he is. They may be much affected by the attitudes taken up by their friends, acquaintances and even strangers in the street. It is clear that all parents suffer at times some unfortunate experience, the unkind remark or the unpleasant look. Much has been done in recent years to help the general public understand the nature of mental handicap. Television, radio programmes, articles in the press, the work of the National Association for Mentally Handicapped Children, are helping to change people's attitudes to the handicapped. The main point is for us all to make some attempt to understand the handicapped, and to treat them as people not very different from ourselves.

Chapter 18

The Future

Bernard has grown up as a full member of our family. At times he has been something of a trial, yet there is a great deal to put on the other side of the balance. Bernard has a pleasant and humorous personality, and has much to contribute to the interest of family life. He is an affectionate child. It has been noticeable that the large number of foreign girls who have helped about our house have all grown very fond of him. Eileen and I, and our other children, have certainly acquired a more varied experience of life through our dealings with Bernard. But what of the future?

We have already described the various ways in which Bernard can work about the house and at the ITU, but of course he has his limitations. For example the following conversation occurred at lunch-time recently between Eileen and Bernard.

'Are your hands clean?'

'Yes.'

'When did you wash them?'

'In David's room.'

'Not where; when?'

'In David's room.'

At this stage Eileen gave up, and Bernard went on eating his lunch, obviously thinking that mum was making very heavy weather of his clean (for once) hands.

We also see his limitations when we try to give him some idea of the use and value of money, so that he will eventually be able to plan the spending of his pocket money. This is not an easy task, because most of his wants are either minimal like an ice cream, or impossible to satisfy like a motor bike or a motor car. However, we made a beginning by suggesting that he save up to buy new batteries for his transistor radio, which ran down at a great rate mainly because of his habit of going to sleep without switching it off. When he wanted a bigger and better transistor, we suggested that he should save up for it. Eileen took him to the shops to find out the cost of new sets, and collected all the relevant catalogues. Then I explained how many weeks' pocket money was involved, and that he would have to wait his time. In due course we bought the set, but we were right to wonder if much of the theory of this operation had sunk in. After a few months he took the set to work with him, without our permission or knowledge, and gave it away to a friend. The first we knew of all this was when the friend's father returned it that evening. Bernard seemed to think that he would be able to go out immediately and buy a new radio. As some sort of reprimand seemed necessary, the radio was placed out of his reach in the lounge for a week!

Although Bernard can be very helpful in and around the house, it must be admitted that he is not an altogether reliable workman. When he is in a good mood, he is as helpful and efficient as his brothers and sister. However, if he does not feel like doing a job, he is not afraid to say so. If Eileen asks him to do something, his most likely reply is 'Andrew, Maureen', and then Eileen has to spell out that they have already done their share. Recently, after watching the news on television, he found a new way of putting over the same point. 'No! Strike.' This at any rate was an amusing variant in an otherwise tedious dialogue.

Just as some supervision is necessary to ensure that tasks are always performed, so some supervision is still necessary to see that he does not do anything silly or dangerous about the house. We do not feel certain that he can deal safely with gas and electricity, and would not like to leave him alone in the house for long, lest he get into some trouble. His bent of mechanical inquisitiveness is only too likely to lead him to fiddle with forbidden appliances if only he gets the opportunity. Periodically we find the record player disturbed by inexpert hands, and recently a film in my camera was mysteriously wound on half a reel. As a result of such experiences, I still make a point of not letting him watch me mend fuses, or see me fill and start our Flymo lawnmower, lest he should attempt these jobs by himself. Similarly, we never leave him alone in the car with the key in the ignition.

Another way in which Bernard needs supervision comes about because he has always shared a bedroom with either Eileen and me or with his brothers or sister. For the past three years he has shared a room with Andrew, and there is a very considerable upset if this routine is disturbed. Last year Andrew was away from home for just under a week, so Bernard was alone in the bedroom. He was very agitated all that week, continually asking 'Andrew home soon?', was reluctant to go to sleep at night, and developed the habit of calling out for mummy. Other rather curious episodes sometimes occur in the middle of the night if he is not feeling well. We occasionally wake up to find that he has gone to the toilet, and then remains standing there, half asleep, and with apparently no idea that it would be sensible to go back to bed. All that is necessary is to lead him back to his room.

Up till now, Bernard has always had his brothers and sister to play with. As David grew older, his place was taken first by Andrew and then by Maureen. At holiday times he plays happily with them all, particularly during the daytime when we are out of doors. They have taught him to play cricket, football and bowls, he can play hide-and-seek, and enjoys a rough and tumble. Indoors, however, it is becoming clear that Bernard is now the youngest of the family and on his own. For example, when we all played paper and pencil games over Christmas we tried to involve Bernard as much as possible in the fetching and carrying of the papers, and he had his books to read, but next day he complained to Eileen that he was bored by these games, and could he watch the television next time.

Although he is now always happy to gaze at television, he is still very weak at amusing himself in other ways. In the past he would cling tenaciously to Eileen whenever she was in the house; there was even a period at the age of about thirteen when he sat outside the door whenever Eileen went to the toilet. He is always ready to look at comics and comic type annuals in bed at night and in the morning, so much so that we sometimes find a whole library in his bed. However, he has always been most reluctant to look at these books in the daytime. Indeed, before Granny came to live with us, there was little that Bernard was willing to do by himself. Nowadays, however, Bernard is only too willing to squat down by the television, and our problem is rather to see that he has some other interests.

Bernard appears quite happy at home at present but time does not stand still. His brothers and sister are growing older, and his granny will not be with us indefinitely. As we have just said, he has few resources for amusing himself, so before very long he may be feeling a need for companionship. At present, the only outside social activity which he could attend is the 7 o'clock club, a joint effort between the ITU and the local branch of the National Society for Mentally Handicapped Children. The club meets once a week at a local community centre, for social evenings, dancing, table tennis, gymnastics, etc. There is also a football team and a sports club which is usually successful at the annual area sports day, its members having won several medals and cups. Apart from this, there is the television, but although we suspect that he would be willing to sit there all day, this does not seem good enough.

Beyond the more immediate problem of seeing that he has adequate interests and companionship, lies the question of what he will do if, as seems quite likely, he lives longer than us. The possible ways of life for the mentally handicapped have changed for better and for worse over the years. In the past, the village idiot had his place in society. There were always simple jobs for an extra pair of hands, and someone to keep an eye on him. However, all this changed with the coming of the industrial revolution. There was no place for him in the new towns and factories. Society did not know what to do with the mentally handicapped, and they became a problem which was not understood. Out of this lack of understanding, there appears to have grown a fear of the unknown, and hence a fear of the handicapped. Certainly by the end of the nineteenth century they were almost all locked up. A typical hospital was an extremely large Victorian building situated out in the country remote from any centre of population. At this time, nearly all mentally handicapped people living in residential institutions were treated in a similar way. The dominant philosophy was that the handicapped could not be trained to do anything useful, or to occupy themselves in a constructive manner; therefore they had to be looked after at as little cost as possible.

Not all that long ago, one local hospital, Borocourt, was very different from what it is today. Visitors arrived once a week by coach from the neighbouring towns. They were admitted through the locked main gate, their bags searched, and their passes checked one by one. There was no question of them visiting the wards. After their passes had been checked, a nurse was sent to bring their relatives from the locked wards to the main hall. Not surprisingly, by the time that the last relative had been produced, it was often time to guide the visitors back into their coach. To complete this picture of a prison-like institution, the inmates wore corduroy trousers, grey blouses and clogs. However, during the last twenty years, a growing number of experiments have shown that even the more severely handicapped can go a long way towards leading a normal life.

Following the Royal Commission of 1954-7 on mental illness and mental deficiency, the Mental Health Act of 1959 provided a completely new basis for the provision of services for both the mentally ill and the mentally handicapped. The emphasis since then has been on encouraging the handicapped, if at all possible, to live either at home or in hostels 'in the community', and to reserve the hospitals for the most severely handicapped. The City of Oxford has built and operates two well-furnished hostels, St Nicholas House for 25 children up to the age of sixteen, and Eastfield House for all older ages. St Nicholas House, the junior hostel, is run mainly on a 5-day week basis, so that the children can return home at weekends and thus maintain links with their parents and relatives, but Eastfield House also provides a permanent home for those whose parents are too old to cope or who have died.

The Health Service envisages that in the future the hospitals will be reserved for the more severely handicapped, i.e. for those much more handicapped than Bernard. However, at present, the hospitals contain many patients basically not more handicapped than Bernard largely because no efforts were made to provide other training and facilities in their earlier years. The principal residential hospital for the area in which we live is the Borocourt Hospital near Reading. The centre of this hospital is a big old mansion set in pleasant parkland. It is surrounded by new buildings, recently completed, which represent a £1 million building programme. These new buildings have been carefully designed for the precise purpose of looking after the mentally handicapped. We were recently conducted round the hospital by the chief nursing officer. There are 600 patients, and he seemed to know the names of all of them, and stopped for a word with most of those we met. It was impossible not to be struck by the high calibre and morale of the staff, and by their great enthusiasm for their jobs. We were impressed by the relaxed attitudes of the patients in the wards and workshops.

The state now provides assistance on a scale much greater than when Bernard was born. Nevertheless, the provision of the services envisaged by the 1959 Act still depends to a great extent on the enthusiasm, or lack of enthusiasm, of particular officers in the local authorities. There is still an urgent need in many areas to increase both the numbers and quality of schools, hostels, hospitals, and other services. It now seems that the public services will make the essential provision for Bernard in the future when this becomes necessary. We are thankful for these services, but they hardly relieve us of a responsibility towards his future security. We believe that he will continue to develop, and will be able to live an active life full of interest for himself, and to make a contribution to his society. However, we also believe that all this will only happen if he continues to live within an atmosphere of affection and love. But how can we ensure this?

The conditions in residential mental hospitals are often far from satisfactory, but we are not entirely happy with the assumption that the handicapped can necessarily be better cared for in small hostels rather than in larger groups. For example, on our visit to Borocourt Hospital we saw the large hall where some social activity is organised every evening, and something of the work of the Friends of Borocourt in providing various amenities for the patients. We gained the impression of an active community where there was always something going on. Borocourt may not be typical of all hospitals, but on the other hand, it is by no means easy to provide comparable activities in a small hostel for only about twenty people of very varied capabilities.

The quality of life for the inmates of a small hostel must depend to a very large extent on the personality of the warden, and this may be a very variable factor. Some hostels show a rapid turn-over of wardens and staff, and also of inmates; in these circumstances the atmosphere can hardly simulate the security of a real home. There is also a very real problem in how the new hostels will provide a full social life for their residents. A hostel built in a town is commonly described as being 'in the community', but this is only a form of words. Unless the residents are easily able to get about, to get to the shops, to church, to the cinema, and to other social functions, they may be as effectively isolated as if they were in the depths of the country. The new methods will only succeed if the hostel is integrated into the community by visits and exchanges on a much more frequent basis than appears usual today.

Another point which must be taken into account is that eventually Bernard will be on his own, without our help to sort out any problems which may arise. It is obvious by reading the press, that there are occasions when the handicapped need expert assistance in dealing with those in authority over them. Indeed there was one episode in Bernard's education when a serious difficulty arose because he was unable to explain fully to us what was happening when he was away from home. It therefore seems necessary to try to arrange for some form of guardianship, either formal or otherwise, so that there will always be someone to take Bernard's part, and to ease his path.

To sum up, we believe that Bernard will continue to develop and will be able to enjoy an active life full of interest for himself, while making a contribution to his society. However, this will only be possible if his environment provides an atmosphere of affection and love. Our present hope is that he will eventually find a home in some form of sheltered community. There is certainly no hurry about this. He is quite happy with us at the moment. However, it may be that he will think differently as he grows older and his brothers and sister leave home. We also feel that if he is going to make such a change that he should make it while he is still young and fairly adaptable, rather than in fifteen or twenty years' time when we suspect that he may have become very set in his ways. However, we trust that reasonable solutions will emerge as the years go by, as indeed they have in the past.

Appendix

Milestones of Progress (Bernard Growing Up)

We here gather together a few details of how Bernard made progress over the years in various important activities.

Eating

Months
6	Takes Farex from a spoon.
9	Drinks from a spoon without dribbling.

Years
1	Tries to drink from a cup.
1¼	Begins on solid food (banana).
1½	Into a high chair.
	Accepts sausage as well as banana.
2	Drinks from a cup without spilling.
	Tries to hold a spoon.
3	Can hold a spoon and pusher.
5	Competent with spoon and fork.
9	Begins to use a knife.
11	Able to cut with a knife.
12	Competent with a knife and fork.

(The corresponding stages for a normal child are of course rather variable. However, we would generally expect him to be drinking from a cup at about 6 months, sitting up in a high chair between 7 and 9 months, and being able to feed himself fairly competently with a knife and fork by the age of 3.)

Toilet training

Years

3	Dry by day and night.
	Clean by day.
5	Clean by day and night.
8	Able to wash hands.
9	Can wash face and bath himself.
11	Dries himself after bath.
	Cleans teeth unsupervised.
12	Baths himself unsupervised.

(The ordinary child is usually clean and dry by day and night at about 3 years of age. Competence in washing comes at about the same time.)

Walking

Years

1½	Sits up unaided.
2	Begins to crawl.
2½	Stands up in play pen.
2¾	First steps.
3½	Learns to go up and down stairs.
4	Running.
5	Walks up a mountain (screaming).
10	Walks up a mountain (sullen).
13	Walks up a mountain (happy).

(The ordinary child generally sits up unaided between 7 and 9 months, begins to crawl and stand up with help between 6 and 12 months, takes his first steps between 12 and 15 months, and goes up and down stairs, possibly crawling, by 18 months.)

Dressing

We list the age when he could first put on various items of clothing.

Years

6	Vest and jumper.
7	Pants.

8	Mitts and socks (heels often at the front).
9	Trousers (right way round).
10	Wellingtons.
11	Sandals on the correct feet with straps fastened.
12	Socks, right way round.
	Gloves.
13	Mackintosh belt.
	Duffle coat and toggles.
14	Ties his tie.

(The normal child learns the easier tasks of dressing between 2 and 3, and the more difficult ones between 4 and 5.)

Talking

Years

3	First word (no).
5	Mama.
7	Dada.
10	Begins to talk comprehensibly (to us).
12	Begins to be understood by family friends.
14	Begins to be understood by strangers.

(An ordinary child generally says 'Mama' at about 9 months and 'no' when he is about 2. From 2 onwards he becomes progressively more fluent and comprehensible.)

Bibliography

The National Association for Mentally Handicapped Children and the National Association for Mental Health publish a number of pamphlets on the problems of mental handicap and the services available. These pamphlets are written in simple terms, and are designed primarily as a first reading for parents and others. The associations also issue lists of books currently available.

The following bibliography gives a brief note on other books which we have found useful. These are written at several levels, some for parents, some for the general public, and others primarily for medical and social workers. Many parents will find something of interest in most of the books, but we have indicated those with a more technical approach by an asterisk. Unless otherwise indicated the place of publication is London.

   (i) Handicapped children
  (ii) Home training
 (iii) School education
  (iv) Learning to talk
   (v) Handicapped adults
  (vi) Community care
 (vii) Residential services
(viii) Medical aspects

(i) Handicapped children

BUCK, PEARL S., *The Child Who Never Grew*, Methuen, 1951. A well-known writer gives an account of her handicapped child. The book chiefly illustrates the strains which may be experienced by parents.

DE VRIES-KRUTT, T., *Small Ship, Great Sea*, Collins, 1971. The story of a mongoloid Dutch boy who died at the age of twenty-five, written by his parents. The book illustrates not only the emotional stresses on the family, but also how much can be achieved with adequate resources, even with a child who was never strong physically.

EGG, MARIA, *When a Child is Different*, Allen and Unwin, 1967. A useful

and sensible book, written for parents, which makes a helpful intro-
duction to the subject. It gives some idea how the child will grow up,
and makes practical suggestions on education and training.

FURNEAUX, B., *The Special Child*, Penguin Books, Harmondsworth, 1969.*
A review of all forms of mental handicap in children and of the provisions for them.

GREEN, MARY, *Elizabeth*, Hodder and Stoughton, 1966. The story of a
mentally handicapped daughter. A moving account by a mother who
could not accept her mongoloid daughter.

HUNT, N., *The World of Nigel Hunt*, Darwen Finlayson, Beaconsfield,
1967. The diary of a mongoloid youth. A fascinating book, although we
ourselves have never met so intelligent a mongol.

KIRMAN, B. H., *The Mentally Handicapped Child*, Nelson, 1972.* A review
written by a psychiatrist to explain the background to mental handicap
and the various types of educational and social services now available.

ROBERTS, NANCY AND BRUCE, *David*, John Knox Press, Richmond, Vir-
ginia, 1968. An interesting book describing a mongol child up to the
age of about 4, with fine photographs of a particularly attractive looking
boy.

VAN DER HOEVEN, J., *Slant-Eyed Angel*, Colin Smythe, Gerrards Cross,
1968. The experience of a father with a mongol son. Mainly about the
parents' reactions to their son.

VAN HOUTEN, NEL, *Bartje, My Son*, Hodder and Stoughton, 1960. The
story of a mentally handicapped son, up to the age of eleven.

(ii) Home training

GEUTER, I., *Adventure in Curative Education*, New Knowledge Books,
East Grinstead, Sussex, 1962. An account of the work of two early
pioneers. It stresses the need for all methods of stimulation, and also
firmness in not letting the child drift.

LOEWY, H., *The Retarded Child*, Staples Press, 1951. A teacher with many
years' experience explains her methods. An old book, but with many
valid lessons.

MOLLOY, J. S., *Teaching the Retarded Child to Talk*, University of London
Press, 1961. Contains much useful and sensible advice on other aspects
of training besides talking.

MORGENSTERN, M. *et al.*, *Practical Training for the Severely Handicapped
Child*, Heinemann Medical Books, 1966. A translation from the original
German book of 1937. Gives good practical advice on methods of
arousing the child's interest.

THEODORE, SISTER MARY, *The Challenge of the Retarded Child*, Bruce,
1963. This book from the USA draws a picture of all levels of retardation.

A sensible and sympathetic book useful as first reading for parents, which also gives practical advice on how to bring up a retarded child.

(iii) School education

GUNZBURG, H. C., *Junior Training Centres*, National Association for Mental Health, 1963. This booklet gives an outline of current principles and methods in schools for the severely handicapped.

GUNZBURG, H. C., *Social Competence and Mental Handicap*, Bailliere, Tindall and Cassell, 1968. Discusses the possibilities of practical social training for retarded children and adolescents leading to a life of partial independence in an open community. Describes the progress charts referred to in chapter 13.

HUTCHINSON, A., *Special Care Units for the Severely Subnormal*, The International League of Societies for the Mentally Handicapped, Brussels, 1967. A pamphlet describing the provisions needed at school to care for children who are both physically and mentally handicapped.

MCDOWALL, E. B., *Teaching the Severely Subnormal*, Edward Arnold, 1964. A handbook for teachers working in the schools.

MARSHALL, A., *The Abilities and Attainments of Children Leaving Junior Training Centres*, National Association for Mental Health, 1967.* The report of a survey to evaluate the effectiveness of school training for the severely handicapped. Very technical.

MINISTRY OF HEALTH, *The Training of Staff of Training Centres for the Mentally Subnormal*, HMSO, 1962. The report of a committee which helped to establish the present pattern of training in the schools.

SEGAL, S. S., *No Child is Ineducable*, Pergamon, 1967. A compendium of information on special education for mentally, physically and socially handicapped children. It includes a large bibliography, and details of the various societies working in this field.

STEVENS, M., *Observing Children who are Severely Subnormal*, Edward Arnold, 1968. A guide to teachers which stresses the need for them to observe their pupils closely. It emphasises the most important points to watch, and the need to keep records.

(iv) Learning to talk

HERMELIN, B. F. and O'CONNOR, N., *Speech and Thought in Severe Subnormality*, Pergamon, 1963.* Experimental studies of the processes of learning to talk.

JOHNSON, W. and MOELLER, D., (eds), *Speech Handicapped School Children*, 3rd ed., Harper and Row, New York, 1967.* An American text quoted as an example of a very negative attitude towards the mentally handicapped (cf. page 337).

LURIA, A. R., *The Role of Speech in the Regulation of Normal and Abnormal Behaviour*, Pergamon, 1961.* The book describes some celebrated Russian experiments which throw light on how the art of speech is acquired by normal children, and the differences which arise in mentally handicapped children.

MOLLOY, J. S., *Teaching the Retarded Child to Talk*, University of London Press, 1961. A good book for parents dealing with speech problems.

(v) Handicapped adults

BARANYAY, E. P., *The Mentally Handicapped Adolescent*, Pergamon, 1971. An account of the Slough Project of the National Society for Mentally Handicapped Children to provide industrial type training for handicapped adolescents.

GUNZBURG, H. C., *Senior Training Centres*, National Association for Mental Health, 1963. A booklet describing the principles and practice of social education and training for older people who are severely handicapped.

INTERNATIONAL LEAGUE OF SOCIETIES FOR THE MENTALLY HANDICAPPED, *Symposium on Sheltered Employment*, Brussels, 1967. The report of an international symposium on how best to provide satisfying work for the handicapped.

NATIONAL SOCIETY FOR MENTALLY HANDICAPPED CHILDREN, *The Pirate Springs Experiment*, 1965. A pamphlet giving an account of a 10-week residential course run by the society to prepare ESN students for outside employment.

NATIONAL SOCIETY FOR MENTALLY HANDICAPPED CHILDREN, *Sexuality and Subnormality*, 1972. A sensible booklet translated from the original edition prepared by the Swedish Board of Health and Welfare.

TUDOR-DAVIES, E. R., *Minimum Intelligence Workers*, National Society for Mentally Handicapped Children, 1968. A pamphlet describing efforts made to enable the less severely handicapped (ESN) to take a job in the outside world.

(vi) Community care

Annual Report of the Medical Officer of Health. A report presented annually to the Health Committee of every local authority in England and Wales. These reports give valuable information on the provisions being made for the mentally handicapped (and on many other matters).

FOTHERINGHAM, J. B., SKELTON, M. and HODDINOTT, B. A., *The Retarded Child and his Family*, Ontario Institute for Studies in Education, 1971. This sound and sensible book describes a Canadian investigation to elucidate the various factors which determine whether a handicapped child is best brought up in his family or in an institution. Although written primarily for social workers and therefore sometimes rather technical, it contains information that many parents may find helpful.

JONES, K., *A History of the Mental Health Services*, Routledge & Kegan Paul, 1972. An interesting account of attitudes to mental handicap and the development of social services to deal with it.

MEYEN, E. L. (ed.), *Planning Community Services for the Mentally Retarded*, International Textbook Co., Scranton, Pennsylvania, 1967. A comprehensive American view of the problems involved, complete with bibliography.

MINISTRY OF HEALTH, *Health and Welfare*, HMSO, 1966. A valuable document which sets out and compares the services for health and welfare, including services for the mentally handicapped, provided by all local authorities in England and Wales.

MINISTRY OF HEALTH, *Report of the Committee on Local Authority and Allied Personal Social Services*, HMSO, 1968. The 'Seebohm Report' surveys the whole field of social services provided by local authorities, and makes recommendations for future developments. It gives an interesting picture of current outlooks on the best ways of caring for the handicapped. A very comprehensive appendix surveys the position of the social services at the time of publication.

NATIONAL SOCIETY FOR MENTALLY HANDICAPPED CHILDREN, *Stress in Families with a Mentally Handicapped Child*, 1967. The report of a working party on the difficulties caused by a handicapped child.

NATIONAL SOCIETY FOR MENTALLY HANDICAPPED CHILDREN, *The Team Approach*, 1971. A report of a seminar to discuss the best methods of integrating medical, social and therapeutic services for the handicapped.

O'CONNOR, N. and TIZARD, J., *The Social Problem of Mental Deficiency*, Pergamon, 1956.* A brief history of earlier methods of treatment followed by a report on the authors' experiments showing how best to train and rehabilitate mentally retarded children.

ROBINSON, K., *Patterns of Care*, National Association for Mental Health, 1961. A lecture by a former minister of health comparing the provision for the handicapped in different foreign countries.

RUTTER, M., TIZARD, J., and WHITMORE, K., *Education, Health and Behaviour*, Longmans, 1970.* Describes a survey of children in the Isle of Wight, and gives detailed information on the incidence of the various types of handicap which call for the provision of public services.

TIZARD, J., *Community Services for the Mentally Handicapped*, Oxford University Press, 1964.* Draws on previous work by the same author to discuss the best way of caring for the mentally handicapped at home and in institutions.

TIZARD, J., and GRAD, J. C., *The Mentally Handicapped and their Families*, Oxford University Press, 1961.* Gives the results of a social survey of the problems of families with a severely subnormal member.

WORLD HEALTH ORGANISATION, *Organisation of Services for the Mentally Retarded*, WHO Technical Report No. 392, 1968. A booklet which reviews the services and sets out the best current practices from different countries.

(vii) Residential services

BARTON, R., *Institutional Neurosis*, John Wright, Bristol, 1966. An interesting but somewhat technical account of the difficulties of maintaining a stimulating atmosphere in an institution.

BRITISH PSYCHOLOGICAL SOCIETY, *Children in Hospitals for the Subnormal*, 1966. A short survey of admissions and educational services.

DEPARTMENT OF HEALTH AND SOCIAL SECURITY, *Better Services for the Mentally Handicapped*, HMSO, 1971. An important paper setting out government policies for the provision of services for the mentally handicapped in the light of modern conditions.

DEPARTMENT OF HEALTH AND SOCIAL SECURITY, *Census of Mentally Handicapped Patients in Hospitals in England and Wales at the end of 1970*, HMSO, 1972. A useful list of the number of patients cared for in the hospitals.

DEPARTMENT OF HEALTH AND SOCIAL SECURITY, *National Health Service Hospital Advisory Service, Annual Report for 1969-70*, HMSO, 1971. The report for this year is primarily concerned with the quality of services for the mentally ill and the mentally handicapped.

DEPARTMENT OF HEALTH AND SOCIAL SECURITY, *Report of the Committee of Inquiry into Allegations of Ill-Treatment of Patients and other Irregularities at the Ely Hospital, Cardiff*, HMSO, 1969. Should be read by everyone interested in the efficient administration of our hospitals.

DEPARTMENT OF HEALTH AND SOCIAL SECURITY, *Report of the Farleigh Hospital Committee of Enquiry*, HMSO, 1971. A report which shows how difficulties can arise in a hospital for the mentally handicapped.

INSTITUTE FOR RESEARCH INTO MENTAL RETARDATION, *Occasional Papers 2, 3 and 4*, Butterworth, 1972.

   Paper 3, 'The need for long-term care' by Sheila Hewett, deals with the factors influencing the decision for a child to live away from home.

   Paper 4, 'Growing up in hospital' by Stephen and Robertson, discusses the modern approach to bringing up children in hospital.

MINISTRY OF HEALTH, *A Hospital Plan for England and Wales*, HMSO, 1962. Details of hospital provision in England and Wales as planned in 1962.

MORRIS, P., *Put Away*, Routledge & Kegan Paul, 1969. A survey of subnormality hospitals which contains much useful and striking information. It suggests that the conditions at the Ely Hospital were not entirely atypical, although it does less than justice to the work going on in the better hospitals.

NATIONAL SOCIETY FOR MENTALLY HANDICAPPED CHILDREN, *Action for the Retarded*, 1971. A conference report, which gives a comprehensive review of the problems of public policy and responsibility in providing residential care.

NATIONAL SOCIETY FOR MENTALLY HANDICAPPED CHILDREN, *Directory of Residential Accommodation for the Mentally Handicapped in England, Wales and N. Ireland*, published periodically. A list of all types of residential accommodation.

STEPHEN, E. (ed.), *Residential Care for the Mentally Retarded*, Institute for Research into Mental Retardation, Pergamon, 1970. The proceedings of a symposium dealing with residential care, which discuss the advantages and limitations of care in hostels and in hospitals.

(viii) Medical aspects

BERG, J. M., (ed.), *Genetic Counselling in Relation to Mental Retardation*, Pergamon, 1971.* A discussion of the basic principles for workers in the field.

CLARKE, A. D. B., *Recent Advances in the Study of Subnormality*, National Association for Mental Health, 1969.* A review of recent professional work written in the first place for the use of medical officers attending courses for mentally subnormal children.

CLARKE, A. M. and CLARKE, A. D. M. (eds), *Mental Deficiency*, 2nd ed., Methuen, 1965.* Probably the best serious treatise on mental handicap. It covers the nature of handicap, its origins, and methods of treatment. Although clearly written it may at times be rather technical for the general reader (like some of the other books in this section). Nevertheless it contains much interesting information.

DOUGLAS, C. P. and HOLT, K. S. (eds), *Mental Retardation: Prenatal Diagnosis and Infant Assessment*, Butterworth 1972.* Technical discussions of prenatal methods of detecting mental handicap and of assessing handicap in 6-month-old babies.

FLEMING, A. C. and PATERSON, H. F., *Mental Disorder and the Law*, E. S. Livingstone, 1969. A booklet summarising those parts of the law relevant to mental handicap.

FRANKS, A. S. T., *Principles and Practice of Dental Care for Patients with Chronic Disease and Disability*, University of Birmingham Dental School, 1960.* A report of a meeting which shows the increasing professional interest in the problem of providing dental treatment for difficult patients, and the quite wide range of attitudes within the profession.

HEATON-WARD, W. A., *Mental Subnormality*, John Wright, Bristol, 1967.* A short handbook of basic information primarily for doctors and nurses.

HILLIARD, L. T., and KIRMAN, B. H. (eds), *Mental Deficiency*, 2nd ed., J. & A. Churchill, 1965.* A comprehensive manual written by distinguished contributors for the professional worker, covering all aspects of mental deficiency.

KIRMAN, B. H., *Mental Retardation*, Pergamon, 1968. A not too technical account of the physical factors responsible for different forms of mental retardation. More useful to workers in the field than to parents concerned only with one form of handicap.

LILLIENFELD, *Epidemiology of Mongolism*, Johns Hopkins Press, Baltimore, 1969.* This book gives a survey of the latest figures for the incidence of mongolism and their association with various factors. A rather technical book.

O'GORMAN, G. (ed.), *Modern Trends in Mental Health and Subnormality*, Vol. I, Butterworth, 1968.* Ten articles covering various aspects of the modern approach to the mentally handicapped including the design and organisation of modern hospitals.

PENROSE, L. S. and SMITH, G. F., *Down's Anomaly*, J. & A. Churchill, 1966.* This book written for doctors gives a comprehensive account of the various aspects, mental and physical, of mongolism (Down's anomaly).

STEVENSON, A. C., 'Applications of chromosome studies in obstetrics and gynaecology', chapter 6 of *Recent Advances in Obstetrics and Gynaecology*, Stallworthy and Bourne (eds), J. & A. Churchill, 1966.* An authoritative account of the relation between mongolism and defects in the chromosomes. Unfortunately rather heavy going for the general reader.

VALENTINE, G. H., *The Chromosome Disorders*, Heinemann Medical Books, 1966.* An up-to-date survey of the various disorders which are now known to arise from aberrations in the chromosomes. Written for doctors, and not very easy reading, but contains some very interesting information.

Index